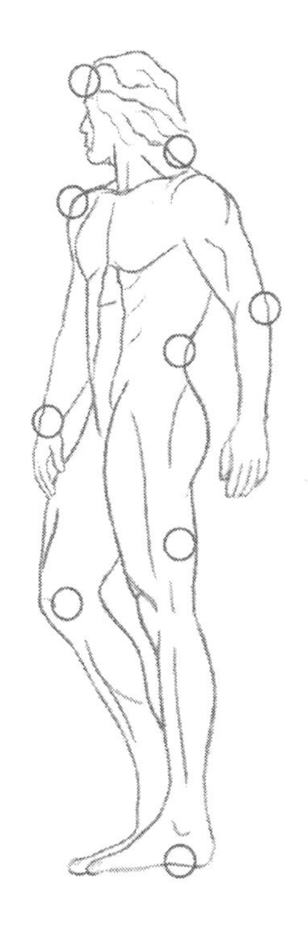

HEALING THE HUMAN MACHINE

Ending spinal, joint and muscular pain.

Dr. Calvin Hargis
Board Certified Chiropractic Orthopedist

Dr. Cal Hargis

Disclaimer

ISBN: 978-1-953773-00-5

Revised: 8/8/2021

Table of Contents

We are powered and held together by nerves, muscles, ligaments, tendons, discs and other forms of soft tissue. When we experience physical pain it is most often due to tearing of these tissues in the form of strains, sprains and other types of trauma. These injuries are seldom improved with massage, heat, vibration or stretch which only increase and prolong our pain. In this book you will learn how to heal soft tissue injuries and end or greatly diminish the pain they produce.

Dr. Cal Hargis

Foreword

While I have a deep respect for the medical profession, few people realize the extremely brief and superficial training medical students receive in the treatment of neck, back, joint and other forms of musculoskeletal (MS) pain. In 2015 only 15% of the 141 medical schools in America mandated training in musculoskeletal diagnosis and treatment with instruction between one and three weeks! This deficient training is wreaking havoc in health care delivery and costing billions of dollars on wasted procedures, tests and prolonged disability.

Specialists like orthopedists and pain management doctors get the same minimal training in medical school and then go on to learn surgical or pharmacological interventions for pain. Seldom do they master how to conservatively evaluate, treat and heal their patients with MS conditions. This lack of substance in medical education has lead to an epidemic of chronic pain sufferers worldwide and has fueled our opioid and heroin crisis in America.

As a result, there is a very high probability that many of the treatments, exercises, postures and methods of relief you currently utilize are dead wrong for your painful condition and keeping you in pain! Back and neck pain, migraines, sciatica, shoulder pain, scoliosis, carpal tunnel and joint complaints are just a few of the musculoskeletal conditions that chronically plague a third of us. In increasing and alarming numbers these same maladies are troubling our children. Could it be that all the advice and therapy you've received has been wrong?

As one of a growing but still small group of chiropractors that are also board certified in orthopedics, I've completed seven years of graduate study in the conservative, non-surgical treatment of musculoskeletal conditions. Combining this with thirty-plus years of clinical experience in treating pain patients one-o-one, I've learned firsthand what does and does not bring relief and cure. My methods have been highly effective without prescriptive medications or surgery. This book will help you achieve similar results.

Books dissecting physical pain can be boring, overly long and wordy, often creating more confusion than clarity. This book won't be one of those. Even complex concepts can be easily understood when presented simply. Inside you will learn in easily understood terms, why you hurt and how to begin getting better today. You'll learn that the most painful conditions are easy to understand and why your prior care either didn't work or didn't last. Unlike other books on the subject, you'll be taught simple tests to evaluate what's causing your pain and the common problems, therapeutic mistakes and bad habits that won't let you heal. You'll also be introduced to the importance of chiropractic evaluation and treatment for spinal and MS complaints. Finally, you will be given the best therapies and the correct postures, exercises and improved body mechanics to begin your recovery. It's as simple as that. Our bodies can heal if we let them.

So, good luck and keep reading. You're about to gain a sane and practical way to reclaim a world filled with personal enjoyment and activity. One last thing, smile... help is on the way.

The Education of a Young Doctor

I had every reason to think I was well prepared when I graduated from chiropractic school. I had just spent the past four years being educated at Palmer, the premier chiropractic college in the US, and had graduated Magna Cum Laude in a large class of aspiring young doctors. My education had been extensive with a curriculum much like medical school in many ways. The difference being, that I knew little of pharmacology but had however received two years of graduate-level training in performing and interpreting x-rays. This also included MRI and CT interpretation. Another significant difference of my chiropractic training and that of a medical doctor was that I spent one-year studying physiotherapy procedures and two years working in a clinic with patients learning the art and science of spinal manipulation under the direction of senior staff advisers.

Fresh out of school and opening my chiropractic office was daunting, especially with three young children and a wife who wanted to be a full-time mom. I began offering the types of care that seemed helpful and patients enjoyed. First, hot packs covered in a thick terry cloth cover would be placed on the patient so they could enjoy ten minutes or so of heat. This would be followed by massage of the painful area which was given by one of my assistants. Finally, I administered gentle manual adjustments to the spine. My patients loved the treatments and my business was booming. I had one problem however; most patients were not making a full recovery. They left the office feeling great but within a couple of days, they were feeling pain again and would be on the phone to reschedule another appointment! For some doctors that would be a win-win situation. For me, caring about making my patients better, it was not.

After a time, I began to see a pattern. When patients presented with neck or lower back pain, the epicenter of their pain was often not in the spine itself, but in the support muscles on either side of the spine. When a patient complained of hip pain, seldom did they point to the hip socket as the source of pain but instead to the muscle tissue in the buttock or upper leg! As a chiropractor, I had been taught to look first to the spine as the source of pain, not the muscle structure. Additionally, when looking at x-rays of my patients who had significant pain, there was often little or no spinal pathology. In many cases when I palpated or probed into the spine there was often less pain than found in the adjacent muscle tissue. That's when I had a minor epiphany: could the majority of pain be due to soft tissue injuries and not spinal issues? And if this was true, could the use of massage and heat keep many of these patients in pain and delay their recovery?

There is a basic concept that seems to have been forgotten by many in the health professions which is simply that the body can heal itself if we allow it to. But if we delay healing by performing the wrong therapies or stressing our injured bodies with the wrong postures can we delay healing perhaps indefinitely? And what is truly damaged in the first place? Yes, many of my patients had spinal pain as a primary condition and required my skillful spinal manipulation to improve. I could stress their spine with any number of orthopedic tests and nerve pain might radiate down a leg or arm. However many of my patients did not have this presentation. Their pain was located in muscle tissue!

This shift in thinking was also at a time just a few years into my practice when I decided to pursue a graduate degree in orthopedics; a three-year journey to learn more. Slowly a diverging concept of pain and injury began to emerge and the logic was inescapable. Our bodies are composed and held together by many 'soft tissues', muscle being by far the most dominant tissue. When we injure ourselves, short of breaking a bone, the only tissue we can injure is soft tissue. In nine out of ten patients I was finding multiple tender points throughout the painful area that clearly indicated muscle injury! It suddenly became apparent that in addition to many legitimate spinal conditions I had also been mistreating a host of soft tissue injuries!

Comprising nearly 45% of our lean body mass, when we injure muscle we seldom experience a complete tear or rupture. Far more commonly we simply strain the muscle, tearing a small percentage of the muscle fibers; fibers that are randomly torn throughout the muscle structure. These diffuse muscle fiber tears create localized inflammation, swelling and pain, so much swelling in fact that we become stiff and tight. As a result, we instinctively stretch, massage, vibrate and heat these damaged areas and it feels so good to do so. But wait; if we have torn fibers within the muscle what is happening when we perform these maneuvers? Well, imagine you have a superficial wound with a nice scab and you rip the scab off! Internal muscle tears are no different. They are simply internal wounds attempting to heal and tissue disruptors like massage and stretch prevent that healing. So why does it feel so good to stretch? Because as you will soon learn, stretching blocks our perception of pain while it heats and loosens injured muscle all the while creating more damage!

This realization, along with my decision to begin the lengthy process of study and examination to become board certified in orthopedics, led me to a gradual 'sea change', in my practice. I completely shifted my emphasis of care. Patients in severe pain started getting better. The ones that needed to come every two or three days started to pace out their appointments as their pain began to lift.

I also began to look at x-rays with a renewed emphasis on structure. Only with standing or ‘weight-bearing’ x-ray studies could one see the full extent of vertebral slippage, spinal joint compressions and abnormal spinal curvatures. Standing x-ray studies became very important in my practice as they could reveal unevenness of the spine due to structural deformities or unequal leg length, major contributors to many forms of acute and chronic pain. I had been taught in my training that spinal pain had to be evaluated from an engineering standpoint because in many cases it was only through the analysis and correction of spinal curvatures and compressions that chronic spinal pain could be resolved. (Medical radiologists do not generally learn or remark on these structural abnormalities.)

I also began to really listen to my patients and learn of their sleep habits, home care and body mechanics to decipher the good from the bad. This coupled with my new approach to treating soft tissue injuries as well as the spine, changed my outcomes significantly and I now saw most patients improving quickly!

I am sad to say, that the changes I made and the therapies I have now been using for the last thirty-odd years have not generally taken hold in this country or most others. On any given day in my clinic, it is common to hear new patients relate their weeks, months or even years of living in chronic pain. They often tell me of their long and unsuccessful journey of seeing multiple doctors and receiving many treatments and tests. I believe there are basic reasons for this, the deficient training of health providers, clinging to old methodology and our primal belief that a tight and painful body part needs to be stretched, massaged and heated.

This book will not solve all your complaints, for the spine is complex, the bio-mechanics of our limbs and movement patterns are complex and many times tissue has been damaged beyond full repair. Therefore this book is not a cure-all and never could be. But the extensive information contained in this book, once understood and applied correctly, has helped thousands of my patients lead happier, more productive and in most cases pain-free lives.

The following pages are somewhat unique in the style they were written. As I take you on a journey of understanding, you will meet patients with complaints identical to yours and see first-hand the methods that worked to alleviate their pain. Since soft tissue injuries are responsible for most acute and chronic pain we will view these brief patient stories from that perspective. As you read their stories most similar to your painful condition, imagine yourself in their place. You will be amazed to find you have been making the same mistakes! Mistakes that are keeping you in pain. You will also learn the many small but important aspects of posture, sleep, nutrition, home care and exercise that will help to make your pain a memory.

In these pages, you will learn all you need to know to have a rational approach to treat acute and chronic pain wherever it may be. Remember though, that no book can see you through a profound injury or a medical emergency. Certain symptoms cannot be taken lightly as I will discuss later under the topic of disc herniations or leg pain. If you have severe, prolonged, unrelenting or worsening pain you need competent medical or chiropractic care to at least rule out a serious underlying problem.

Much of this book is dedicated to the healing of soft tissue injuries. However one can't dismiss the importance of a healthy non-compromised spine that fully emits spinal nerve flow to ensure proper function to every bodily organ. In that regard chiropractic care is a must for good health. Spinal manipulation can resolve and prevent a host of health issues and later we will take a closer look at the many benefits of spinal hygiene and chiropractic spinal manipulation.

Now let's take a look at the sad state of affairs that surrounds acute and chronic pain treatment in the world today and some of the reasons why.

Treating Pain: Cracks in the System

In a five-year study performed by researchers from the Mayo Clinic of 142,377 residents of Olmsted County, Minnesota over 55% of doctor visits were for joint problems or back pain.

Pain the Epidemic

Chronic pain is America's greatest health problem. Usually defined as pain lasting more than three months, chronic pain affects 100 million adult Americans, according to a 2011 report from the National Academy of Sciences' Institute of Medicine. In 2011, that was nearly 40% of the adult population. Chronic pain is the leading reason people go to doctors and it costs the nation over $635 billion a year; more than cancer, heart disease and diabetes combined. Back pain alone is the leading cause of disability in Americans under 45 years of age. More than 26 million Americans between the ages of 20 and 64 years of age experience frequent back pain impacting every facet of their lives.

If you have back or other chronic pain your chances of getting better are poor! A study conducted by Barlow and colleagues, for the Center for Health Studies of Seattle, Washington, and published in ‘Spine’, a leading periodical for physicians, shocked many with their findings. They interviewed 1,128 recent and longer-term back pain patients one year after seeking treatment with primary care physicians. Sixty-nine percent of the acute pain patients and eighty-two percent of the chronic back pain patients were still experiencing back pain![1]

Another study by Drs. T. H. and E. K. Hansson also published in Spine, interviewed 2,080 men and women in Denmark, Germany, the Netherlands, Sweden, Israel and the United States. Each had been disabled with chronic pain for at least ninety days. They were interviewed at three months, one year and at a two-year follow-up. Patients had a choice of health care treatments that were similar in all countries. The results however, were surprisingly the same! The study concluded that "Almost none of the commonly occurring and frequently practiced medical interventions for patients who are sick-listed because of low back pain had any positive effects on either the recorded health measures or work resumption."[2]

Pain STORY (Pain Study Tracking Ongoing Responses for a Year), a UK Medical Press Release Dated August 2009, tracked patients with chronic pain over one year. These patients experienced chronic musculoskeletal (MS) pain; spinal pain of the neck and back, arthritis, headache, nerve pain and mixed pain. They followed them for one year to gauge their improvement. To qualify the patients had to have been in pain for at least three months at a moderate to severe, 5 to 10, pain score on a 10 point pain scale where 0 indicated no pain and 10 the worst pain imaginable. The findings were startling; despite medical and other treatments, 95% of the patients continued to suffer from moderate to severe chronic pain. 56% of the patients' pain levels failed to improve during a year's treatment and 19% of them got worse![3] These studies have been duplicated many times.[4]

28,000 working adults, surveyed in the American Productivity Audit found that 52.7% of the workforce reported headaches, back pain, arthritis or other musculoskeletal pain in the prior two weeks with 12.7% absent from work or with diminished capacity in the same period! (Lost productivity due to musculoskeletal conditions are estimated to cost $61.2 billion per year to employers.)

A 2006 survey commissioned by the American Pain Foundation found that more than half of chronic pain sufferers felt they had little or no control over their pain. They reported experiencing breakthrough pain one or more times daily severely impacting their quality of life and overall well-being. More than three-quarters of chronic pain patients felt depressed. Almost three-quarters said they had trouble concentrating and had low energy levels. Eighty percent reported an inability to sleep well.

While many studies ignore children and adolescents they should not. Our children are quickly swelling the ranks of the afflicted as they struggle with massive book bags and have their very real complaints superficially dismissed as 'growing pains'. These statistics are disturbing but not as disturbing as what comes next.

America... Drug Nation

America has a problem and it started long ago. As a child of the '50s watching our first black and white TV, the ad I remember above all others was the Alka Seltzer ad; "Plop-plop, fizz-fizz, oh what a relief it is!" With those first subtle messages, Americans and indeed much of the world were being conditioned and groomed to adopt a new way of thinking; if you want to feel better you need a pill. With time and the billions spent on similar advertising, we as a nation have been shaped to believe that health and a quick fix comes in a bottle. No longer do we have to take personal responsibility for our health; we can eat what we want, drink to excess and lounge on the couch. It's all good. We have meds for high blood pressure, diabetes and gout. We have gastric bypass for the fat, miracle drugs for our cancers and open-heart surgery for the sludge in our arteries! Between 1986 and 2002 Americans age 45 and older reported their regular use of prescription drugs increased from 52% to 75%. On average, people aged 45 and older say they take four prescription medications daily.[5]

But now we have a real crisis. According to the National Institute of Health, although Americans make up just 4% of the world population, at the end of the last decade, they were consuming 83% of the world's total OxyContin supply each year and 99% of the world's hydrocodone supply! This wave of abusive prescribing and consumption has evolved into our present day heroin epidemic. Both OxyContin and heroin are opiates and use between the two is highly linked. Many people who begin abusing opioids to the point of addiction run out of their supply. Often they turn to a similar drug like heroin that's cheaper and easier to obtain. Using OxyContin makes a person 19 times more likely to use heroin in their lifetime, according to the National Institute on Drug Abuse for Teens.

Drug overdoses in America now exceed 220,000 thousand each year and roughly 70,000 result in death! According to the National Survey on Drug use and Health, 21.5 million Americans (aged 12 and older) battled a substance use disorder in 2014. Drug abuse and addiction costs American society close to $200 billion in healthcare provision, criminal justice administration and lost workplace production/participation according to the Office of National Drug Control Policy.

How did we get into this mess? In the 1990s, opioids were heavily marketed by drug companies for moderate to severe chronic pain management.[6] Drug companies also minimized the addictive risks of these medications to prescribing physicians.[7] Overworked and uncertain, many doctors turned to heavily touted opioids to control pain. Unfortunately, (as you will soon learn), many health providers were and continue to be, so poorly trained to evaluate and treat such complaints that they had little understanding of how to proceed. In their confusion, they turned to more pain control. Primary care physicians accounted for the largest volume of prescriptions for opioid medications.[8,9] Between 2007 and 2012, the opioid-prescription rate grew exponentially among family practice, general practice and internal medicine specialties.[10] Most (but not all) of the doctors prescribing these drugs were well-intentioned, not meaning to create addicts. They simply didn't have the training to pursue a better course of care.

Millions of addicts have created another problem. Studies indicate that less than 20% of primary care physicians consider themselves "very prepared to identify alcohol or drug dependence." This contrasts with more than 80% feeling very comfortable diagnosing hypertension and diabetes.[11] "Both pain medicine and addiction have gotten short shrift in medical school, but of the two, addiction has received much less attention," states Anna Lembke, MD, director of the addiction medicine fellowship and assistant professor of psychiatry and behavioral sciences at Stanford University in California. Medical students learn more about addiction now than they did 20 years ago, "but not much more," she said. "A silver lining of the opioid epidemic, if one can be found, is that medical schools are more interested than ever in teaching how to screen and intervene for addiction, particularly opioid use.[12]

When the Experts Aren't So Expert

Most people with back pain see their medical doctor. It seems like a logical move when one considers the advances of modern medicine. Well brace yourself: your typical, dedicated and caring M.D., possesses little skill or training in the diagnosis and treatment of back pain or the care of other painful musculoskeletal (MS) conditions! In 2007, C.S. Day, along with other researchers surveyed Harvard medical student's competence in performing musculoskeletal physical examinations. Only 26% of the fourth year students passed a validated MS examination! These students cited insufficient curriculum time devoted to musculoskeletal education as the reason.[13]

Between 2014-2015, B. F. DiGiovanni and colleagues collected information from all of the 141 US medical schools. They wanted to gauge the depth of training imparted to medical students in the diagnosis and treatment of musculoskeletal conditions. They found that instruction in this area was mandated for between one and up to three weeks in only 15% of the schools! Other schools offered short courses to students on an elective or optional basis![14] They titled their study, 'Musculoskeletal Medicine Is Underrepresented in the American Medical School Curriculum.'

In 2015 a study was published by Weiss and colleagues of an examination given to 405 medical students to determine their competency in musculoskeletal medicine. The results appeared in the February 2015, American Journal of Orthopedics. The average examination score was a meager 40 on a 100 point scale, far below passing. UCLA's Dr. Andrew Charles, who runs the Headache Research and Treatment Programs at the David Geffen School of Medicine states, "Medical schools should do a better job of preparing physicians to identify and treat chronic pain."

The typical MD has little training in determining the underlying cause of your musculoskeletal pain or the beneficial versus harmful therapies applicable to your particular condition. Further, few have knowledge of the role that poor body mechanics or poor postural habits have in stressing your body and prevent healing. (When is the last time your medical doctor asked about your sleep position? This is a topic critical for the recovery from back pain). With little hands-on experience in the care and rehabilitation of pain patients, most M.D.'s depend largely on a wide battery of prescription drugs to alleviate pain.

While it may seem barbaric, pain can be a good thing since it is a barometer of injury and improvement! Pain also lets us know which habits, postures and therapies are helpful or hurtful. Very strong medications like opioids may numb us so severely that we can injure ourselves more in our desensitized state.

Prescribed drugs don't cure but only numb pain and when symptoms continue, the next step usually is expensive and extensive high tech testing: MRI, CT and electro-diagnostic nerve testing. This produces two types of very popular but faulty medical thinking: If the problem can't be imaged by a multi-million dollar MRI machine it doesn't exist. This is unfortunate since many soft tissue injuries are not visualized by MRI. Conversely, many preexisting structural problems may be seen on MRI, such as old disc protrusions or herniations. Many times these may be falsely targeted as the source of pain and leads to a non-productive and often risky surgery!

If the tests turn out negative the treatment of choice for millions experiencing continued spinal pain is more medication! That's right, an approach largely ineffective with side effects that can undermine one's health and produce risky interactions with other drugs taken in combination. This is a solution that does little to resolve spinal pain but is likely to make you drug dependent on opioids or other meds. It does however line the pockets of pharmaceutical companies and insures your frequent visitation and dependence on your M.D.!

Since the cradle, we've all been conditioned to desire fast pain relief. This thinking may be great for an upset stomach but musculoskeletal pain is generated from injury or biomechanical stress and requires competent treatment and time to heal. Unfortunately, medications offer only short-term relief, lasting only as long as the drug is in your system, having done little to address the underlying pathology producing pain.

Another option for pain relief might be physical therapy. An option usually made when pain responds poorly to medication, lingers or is severe. However since we have seen that your primary care physician may know little about the nature and source of your pain, their prescriptions for therapy can do more harm than good! Moreover, the M.D. can also dispense an 'evaluate and treat accordingly script' thus leaving the choice of treatment up to the physical therapist. In my experience, physical therapists take their title quite seriously. Often their treatment of patients is too physical. The use of stretching, massage and overly forceful exercise disrupts healing soft tissues that are still very fragile. This can result in greater tissue injury, leaving the patient with increased pain and impairment. (To be fair, I have found physical therapists to be fantastic at performing rehab for many conditions and especially after shoulder, hip, knee or other forms of surgery.)

What about the orthopedic specialist? Certainly, the orthopedist is specialized with years of advanced training to acquire and perfect their surgical skills. But since the vast majority of musculoskeletal (MS) pain sufferers don't warrant surgery are they more skilled in conservative treatment? Orthopedists have the same basic and deficient MS training in medical school and then go on to learn the surgical interventions particular to their craft. Seldom do they work closely with patients performing conservative non-surgical therapies or methods of treatment.

The bottom line is that few general medical practitioners today can accurately identify the exact nature of MS pain! In seeing multiple doctors, patients may receive as many varying opinions as to the nature of their pain, while thousands of dollars of expensive and often contradictory testing may be ordered. No wonder confusion reigns in the treatment of pain! When you couple this with the fact that typically your medical doctor hasn't been trained to read x-rays but relies on a radiologist's report, things can go from bad to worse. As you will later see, radiologists often fail to recognize or comment on the most basic structural problems revealed on x-ray!

Overtreating Back Pain… a Profitable Business

The prevalence of spinal pain hasn't increased much in the past twenty years. About a quarter of Americans report back pain in any three months.[15] Despite this, a whole universe of expensive diagnostic tests and treatments has arrived. Injections, surgical procedures, implantable devices and new pain medications are growing at an alarming rate. These tests and procedures are needed for some patients but their use has expanded beyond their need or clinical indication. This is largely being driven by a litigious society, professional concern, marketing and greed.[16,17]

The development of new drugs and devices for the treatment of spinal and other forms of musculoskeletal (MS) pain has outpaced the scrutiny of their use and worth. Complications and death related to pain management are increasing. This is happening as the confidence in new drugs and devices is eroding by revelations of misleading advertising, allegations of kickbacks to physicians and major investments by surgeons in the products they endorse![18,19,20,21,22]

Magnetic resonance imaging (MRI) is just one example. MRI scanning for the lumbar spine is recommended to be used judiciously and recommended only for severe and prolonged pain, weakness, or functional impairment of the legs, bladder or bowel. Nevertheless, MRI imaging has increased in the Medicare population by over 300% in the last decade or so. Surgery rates are highest where imaging rates are highest. When the number of studies performed is compared to the indications for their use, two-thirds of these MRI's may be inappropriate. Why so many? Fearful patients demand it, doctors want it for diagnostic purposes (also as a protection from litigation) and lastly... it's a money maker.[23,24,25,26,27]

If you're in pain the biggest problem with imaging is that it may lead to false conclusions about the origin of your pain. Positive findings, including herniated disks that could have been present for months or years, are common in asymptomatic people and just because they're found in those with pain doesn't mean they're the cause. In a study of sixty-seven individuals, who didn't have or never had low-back pain or sciatica, lumbar MRI scans were performed. The MRIs were interpreted independently by three neuro-radiologists who had no knowledge concerning the lack of symptoms by the participants. About one-third of the subjects were found to have a substantial abnormality. Of those below sixty years of age, 20% had a herniated disc and one had spinal stenosis (narrowing of the spinal canal). In the group above sixty, 57 of the scans showed either herniated discs or spinal stenosis. 35% of the subjects between twenty and thirty-nine years had disc pathology as did all but one of the sixty to eighty-year-old subjects. Given the positive MRI findings often seen in asymptomatic subjects, any abnormalities on an MRI should be looked at somewhat skeptically and should be strictly correlated with age and any clinical signs and symptoms before operative treatment is contemplated.[28]

Surgery isn't necessarily the answer either. In a study appearing in the Journal of Bone and Joint Surgery, 495 patients with disc-related back pain presented for surgical consultation in the offices of 16 different surgeons. Eighty-six patients had surgery within 6 months of enrollment. Surgery consisted of instrumented fusion (using metal straps and screws to secure two or more spinal vertebrae together) 79%, disc replacement (with an artificial disc) 12%, laminectomy (removal of spinal bone) or discectomy (partial disc removal) 9%. The majority of the 495 patients received no surgery. Surgery showed only a minor benefit over nonsurgical treatment on follow-up disability questionnaires one year later. The success rate was 33% for surgery and 15% for nonsurgical treatment. The rate of re-operation was 11% in the surgical group. Only 6% of those patients who were in the non-surgical group received surgery at 12 months after enrollment. While the surgical group showed greater improvement at 1 year compared with the nonsurgical group, the composite success rate for both treatment groups was only fair.[29]

Researchers reviewed the records of 1,450 patients in the Ohio Bureau of Worker's Compensation database who had a diagnosis of disc degeneration, disc herniation and/or radiculopathy with tingling, pain or numbness radiating into the leg. A total of 725 surgeries for lumbar fusion were compared to 725 control subjects who had equivalent pain but did not have surgery. Two years after fusion surgery, 26% of the fusion cases had returned to work (RTW), whereas 67% of the nonsurgical controls were back at work! The re-operation rate was 27% for surgical patients. Of the lumbar fusion subjects, 36% had complications related to the surgery! Permanent disability rates were 11% for the surgery cases and 2% for those avoiding the knife. For the lumbar fusion group, daily opiate use increased 41% after surgery. The total number of days off from work was averaged at 1,140 for the surgical fusion group as compared to 316 days for the non-surgical group. It was concluded that lumbar fusion for the diagnoses of disc degeneration, disc herniation, and/or radiculopathy is associated with a significant increase in disability, opiate use, prolonged work loss and poor RTW status.[30]

Another study looked at 100 patients who underwent instrumented spinal fusion for persistent back and/or leg pain that had lasted more than 1 year despite one or more previous spine surgeries. All patients underwent medal strap and screw fixation with a spinal fusion of one or more vertebrae. After a mean follow-up period of 15 months, 35% of the patients reported a good outcome, whereas 65% had unsatisfactory outcomes. The study showed disappointing results in terms of perceived recovery, functional disability and pain. It was determined that conservative (non-surgical) management was more beneficial and therefore suggests that more selective and careful assessment should be done to prevent unnecessary surgery.[31]

Surgeries like lumbar fusion are usually prompted by chronic back pain and many patients receive long-term preoperative opioid analgesics. In the medical journal Pain, Dr. R. Deyo and colleagues did a study to determine the number of long-term preoperative opioid users that discontinued or reduced their dosage after surgery. The study included 2491 adults undergoing lumbar fusion surgery for degenerative conditions. 1045 patients had received long-term opioids before their surgeries. They found that 77.1% continued long-term postoperative use of these medications after surgery and 13.8% continued episodic use. Only 9.1% discontinued or had short-term postoperative use. Among preoperative users, 34.4% received a lower dose postoperatively, but 44.8% received a higher long-term dose! Among patients with no preoperative opioids, 12.8% became long-term users.[32]

Finally, a retrospective analysis reported on 69 patients twelve years after having an uncomplicated lumbar disc surgery in order to evaluate degenerative changes and segmental instability at these disc levels. Two independent radiologists evaluated the patients' lumbar x-rays in various endpoints of movement. The results were shocking; degenerative changes and segmental instability were significantly more frequent in operated than non-operated lumbar segments! Their conclusion; lumbar disc surgery was associated with an increased risk of degeneration and segmental instability in the long term.[33]

The Downward Spiral

Chronic back pain sufferers may receive medications for years or a lifetime as they spiral ever downward in their functional levels. They become increasingly dependent on a dangerous cocktail of drugs to combat pain, sleeplessness, fatigue, anxiety and depression. Chronic pain is exhausting to the body as it leads to....

- fears concerning job security and our ability to provide financial support for our families
- images of deeper problems producing our pain such as organ disease or cancer
- sleep deprivation
- depression and anxiety as we begin to view our lives within the context of diminishing potentials
- secondary body pain affecting the shoulders, hips, knees, elbows or other body areas may develop as we become deconditioned and subject to movement patterns as we try to avoid pain
- withdrawal from life itself as we are beset by despair, embarrassment and resentment by and of family, friends and a medical establishment that has few answers and often little empathy

Medical and Chiropractic Care

Chiropractors look at the body holistically; one perfect and integrated self-healing entity with an innate capacity to maintain health. Rest, exercise, best nutrition, positive spirit and an unimpeded and non-compromised nervous system are essential to this end. Medical doctors tend to look at each malady or disease of the human body as a unique entity; diabetes requiring this list of medications, high blood pressure another and so on. There's nothing wrong with combating illness. But when you treat each condition with medications, many of which have side effects as bad potentially as the entity being treated and often at a cost that can literally bankrupt the patient, maybe the pendulum of health care has gone slightly off-kilter. Perhaps it needs to swing in a more natural direction with an emphasis on maintaining a healthier lifestyle rather than 12th-hour interventions.

Why See a Chiropractor?

A growing number of satisfied patients might tell you to visit a chiropractor. Doctors of chiropractic, (D.C.'s), are seen by approximately fifty million Americans for the treatment of back pain, headaches, sciatica or various other painful conditions. They have a good reason for making such a choice. After spending years at the undergraduate level with a heavy science concentration, chiropractors receive four additional years of training focusing on the diagnosis and treatment of the spine and musculoskeletal system. Their instruction in the area of conservative spinal treatment is rigorous and complete, far exceeding that of either medical or physical therapy schools.

Another strong fact to consider is that I, like most chiropractors, cannot prescribe medications to lessen or mask pain. This means that unlike the M.D. a D.C. has little room for error in determining what's causing your pain or how to fix it. We either get results or our patients walk!

Another unique feature of chiropractic training is that all chiropractic students spend two or more years learning to take and interpret x-rays and as well as other forms of advanced imaging. Chiropractors are required to read x-ray, CT and MRI studies for pathology. M.D.'s only receive such training if they specialize in radiology or advanced specialties like orthopedics! More importantly, chiropractors look at spinal x-rays using engineering principles and spinal measurements to determine the positioning, structure and integrity of the spine and its many components.

The spine is composed of twenty-four movable vertebrae subject to injury or growth abnormality and is balanced atop the pelvis and lower extremities which may present with structural problems of their own. Solving spinal pain is complex. The chiropractic physician's true value is his or her ability to evaluate and effectively treat these complexities. In many cases, the identification of abnormal spinal mechanics and corrective treatment of these conditions is the only way to resolve spinal pain and nerve pain generated from the spine. Medical radiologists have little training in the evaluation of spinal mechanics and seldom discuss or disclose these issues in their reports. It is a terrible misfortune that these abnormalities are never addressed for they are responsible for spinal pain and much suffering. More will be said about this later in the book.

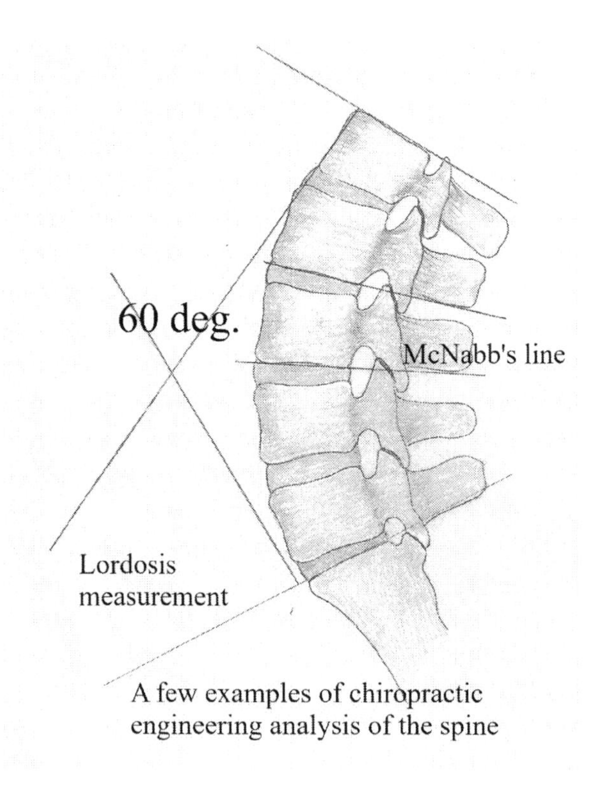

A few examples of chiropractic engineering analysis of the spine

After having identified one or more spinal issues chiropractors employ healing therapies, tailored exercise programs, nutritional counseling, orthotic or brace application, ergonomic and postural recommendations and spinal manipulation as needed. If spinal manipulation is indicated your chiropractor is well trained in this area. Chiropractors receive at least three years of instruction in spinal manipulation, which as you will later see, is considered a safe and effective therapy. (Some physical therapists receive very limited instruction in spinal manipulation and should not perform spinal manipulation in my opinion and experience.)

Chiropractic treatment also carries an exceptional endorsement contained in "Acute Low Back Pain in Adults: Assessment and Treatment", a report released by the U.S. Department of Health and Human Services (HHS). HHS had asked a group of twenty-three distinguished physicians and specialists to examine the growing crisis of low back pain in America and to make recommendations about care. For many months they looked at outcomes of various forms of care for low back pain. The recommendations by the panel, most of whom were medical doctors, shocked much of the health care industry. They found that the majority of care for acute low back pain was of little worth! This included forms of therapy like stretching and massage! What did they recommend? Chiropractic care.[34] Sound surprising? Not if you're one of the millions of Americans who regularly see a chiropractor.

Chiropractic Manipulation; the Risk Myth

According to the Cunningham Group who advertise as malpractice insurance specialists, the average cost of malpractice insurance for medical doctors in my geographic area of practice which is Orange County, New York is as follows; $16,163.00 for general practitioners or family physicians, $124,970.00 for surgeons and $172,874.00 for OB/GYN doctors. As a chiropractor, I currently pay less than $2000.00 per year in premiums. Since injury risk determines malpractice rates you can quickly see that chiropractic care is considered very safe.

Some medical professionals have overstated the possibility of stroke following cervical manipulation of the spine. Numerous studies have refuted this. Since the first signs of stroke are often neck pain and headaches days or weeks before the actual event, many patients may visit a chiropractor for these symptoms prior to having the stroke and manipulation has been falsely blamed.

Serious complications following spinal manipulative therapy (SMT) of the cervical spine, including stroke, are rare. Dr. Keith Overland, past president of the American Chiropractic Association, has stated that because of their high degree of training and specificity of spinal manipulation Chiropractors apply forces in manipulation that are, "no greater than people normally achieve in activities of daily life." Dr. Scott Haldeman MD et al reviewed a full 10 years' worth of malpractice claims files in Canada for the 4500 chiropractors in practice. They found that the likelihood that chiropractic manipulation would result in stroke was 1 per 5.85 million cervical adjustments![35] A second study by J. D. Cassidy and colleagues reviewed 9 years of Ontario Hospital Records and concluded that there was no evidence of excess risk of stroke associated with chiropractic care as compared to primary medical care.[36]

Now let's take a critical look at the safety of medicine. Dr. Lucian Leape, a researcher at the Harvard Medical School of Public Health, states that only 13-15% of medical procedures have ever been tested for appropriateness by randomized trials. He notes that medical care results in adverse events in 3.7 percent of all hospitalizations. Worse yet, 13.6 percent of these adverse events lead to death. He states: "Medicine is now a high-risk industry, like aviation. But, the chance of dying in an aviation accident is one in two million, while the risk of dying from a medical accident is one in two hundred!"[37]

The most comprehensive review of adverse events by modern medicine was the study reported in "Death by Medicine", co-authored by Gary Null Ph.D., Carolyn Dean M.D., N.D., Martin Feldman, M.D., Debora Rasio, M.D. and Dorothy Smith, Ph.D. Published in 2003 and 2004 their data was collected from close inspection of medical peer-reviewed journals and government statistics.

This fully referenced report reveals that:

2.2 million people experience in-hospital, adverse reactions to prescribed drugs per year.

20 million unnecessary antibiotics are prescribed annually for viral infections

7.5 million unnecessary medical and surgical procedures are performed annually, and

8.9 million people are exposed to unnecessary hospitalization every year!

The most stunning statistic however, was the total number of deaths caused by conventional medicine; an astounding 783,936 per year! That is a mind-boggling 2147 people killed daily! In the words of the researchers, "It is now evident that the American medical system is the leading cause of death and injury in the US." (By contrast, the number of deaths attributable to heart disease in 2001 was 699,697, while the number of deaths attributable to cancer was 553,251.)[38]

There is no doubt that modern medicine in America and the developed countries, is in many ways miraculous and has saved countless lives, just as it has saved mine and more than once. But one must be aware that no system is perfect and the biggest advocate for your health is you, the wise consumer. The biggest determinate of your health is the care and feeding of your own human machine.

Now let's look at some studies on the effectiveness of chiropractic care.

Research Studies Concerning Chiropractic

In the Journal of Manipulative and Physiological Therapeutics, May 2000, researchers looked at the one-month outcomes of patients seeing either M.D.s or D.C.s. Chiropractors far outpaced medical doctors in patient satisfaction. On average chiropractic patients showed impressive improvement: a 31% reduction in pain severity and a 29% reduction in disability reduction. Patients also demonstrated a 36% improvement in sensory pain quality and 57% in affective pain quality. Medical patients showed a minimal improvement in pain severity by 6% and functional disability by 1%. The medical patients actually demonstrated deterioration in sensory perception of pain by 29% (location, quality and intensity) and diminished emotional outlook with increased negativity and depression by 26%.[39]

Another interesting study by Croft and colleagues looked at the outcomes of 490 men and women treated for low back pain by

M.D.s. Sampled one year later 75% of these patients were still experiencing back pain.[40]

A 1998 study by Drs. Konrad, Curtis, Smucker and Carey, which appeared in the 'Archives of Family Medicine', interviewed 189 physicians, chiropractors and their patients both initially after the first office visit and then six months later. There were striking differences between self-confidence scores of physicians and chiropractors; 42% of physicians felt poorly prepared to manage low back pain when they first entered practice, compared with only 15% of chiropractors. Furthermore, the chiropractic patients reported dramatically higher levels of satisfaction with their treatment and response than did those individuals treating with an M.D.[41]

Kazis and colleagues found that patients who saw a chiropractor as their initial provider for low back pain (LBP) had a 90% decrease in their odds of both early and long-term opioid use.[42]

Dr. Cristine Goertz and her research team found chiropractic manipulative therapy in conjunction with standard medical care offered a significant advantage for decreasing pain and improving physical functioning when compared with only standard care, for men and women between 18 and 35 years of age with acute low back pain.[43]

In a randomized controlled trial conducted by Dr. Korthal-de-Bos, 183 patients with neck pain were randomly allocated to manual therapy (spinal mobilization), physiotherapy (mainly exercise) or general practitioner care (counseling, education and drugs) in a 52-week study. The clinical outcomes measures showed that manual therapy resulted in faster recovery than physiotherapy and general practitioner care. Moreover, the total cost for the patients receiving chiropractic therapy was about one-third of the cost of physiotherapy or general practitioner care.[44]

In Other Studies

Patients with chronic low-back pain treated by chiropractors showed greater improvement and satisfaction at one month than patients treated by family physicians. Satisfaction scores were higher for chiropractic patients. A higher proportion of chiropractic patients (56 percent vs. 13 percent) reported that their low-back pain was better or much better, whereas nearly one-third of medical patients reported their low-back pain was worse or much worse.[45]

The results of a clinical trial showed that chiropractic care combined with usual medical care for low back pain provides greater pain relief and a greater reduction in disability than medical care alone. The study, which featured 750 active-duty members of the military, is one of the largest comparative effectiveness trials between usual medical care and chiropractic care ever conducted.[46]

Manual-thrust (spinal) manipulation provides greater short-term reductions in self-reported disability and pain compared with usual medical care. 94% of the manual-thrust manipulation group achieved greater than 30% reduction in pain compared with 69% of usual medical care.[47]

Reduced odds of surgery were observed for those whose first provider was a chiropractor. 42.7% of workers [with back injuries] who first saw a surgeon had surgery, in contrast to only 1.5% of those who first saw a chiropractor.[48]

Acute and chronic chiropractic patients experienced better outcomes in pain reduction, improved functional ability and patient satisfaction; clinically important differences in pain and disability improvement were found for chronic patients.[49]

In a randomized, controlled trial, researchers compared the effectiveness of manual therapy (spinal adjustments), physical therapy, and continued care by a general practitioner (M.D.) in patients with nonspecific neck pain. The success rate at seven weeks was twice as high for the manual therapy group (68.3 percent) as for the continued care group (general practitioner). Manual therapy scored better than physical therapy on all outcome measures. [50]

Cervical spine manipulation was associated with significant improvement in headache outcomes in trials involving patients with neck pain and/or neck dysfunction and headache.[51]

Four weeks after the cessation of treatment, patients who had received cervical spine manipulative therapy (for episodes of severe headache), experienced a sustained therapeutic benefit in all major outcomes in contrast to the patients that received amitriptyline therapy, who had little to no relief.[52]

In a study funded by NIH's National Center for Complementary and Alternative Medicine to test the effectiveness of different approaches for treating mechanical neck pain, 272 participants were divided into three groups that received either spinal manipulative therapy (SMT) from a doctor of chiropractic (DC), pain medication (over-the-counter pain relievers, narcotics and muscle relaxants) or exercise recommendations. After 12 weeks, about 57 percent of those who had chiropractic care and 48 percent who exercised reported at least a 75 percent reduction in pain, compared to 33 percent of the people in the medication group. After one year, approximately 53 percent of the drug-free groups continued to report at least a 75 percent reduction in pain; compared to just 38 percent pain reduction among those who took medication.[53]

Findings from a study utilizing data from the North Carolina State Health Plan collected between 2000-2009 show that care by a doctor of chiropractic (DC) alone or DC care in conjunction with care by a medical doctor (MD) was much more cost effective for uncomplicated lower back pain than MD care with or without care by a physical therapist.[54]

Older Medicare patients with chronic low back pain and other medical problems who received spinal manipulation from a chiropractic physician had lower costs of care and shorter episodes of back pain than patients in other treatment groups. Patients who received a combination of chiropractic and medical care had the next lowest Medicare costs and patients who received medical care only incurred the highest costs.[55]

Low back pain initiated with a doctor of chiropractic (DC) saves 20 to 40 percent on health care costs when compared with care initiated through a medical doctor (MD), according to a study that analyzed data from 85,000 Blue Cross Blue Shield (BCBS) beneficiaries in Tennessee over a two-year span. The study population had open access to MDs and DCs through self-referral, and there were no limits applied to the number of MD/DC visits allowed and no differences in co-pays. Researchers estimated that allowing DC-initiated episodes of care would have led to an annual cost savings of $2.3 million for BCBS of Tennessee. They also concluded that insurance companies that restrict access to chiropractic care for low back pain treatment may inadvertently pay more for care than they would if they removed such restrictions.[56]

Researchers analyzing the prevalence, patterns and predictors of chiropractic utilization in the U.S. general population found that, "Back pain and neck pain were the most prevalent health problems for chiropractic consultations and the majority of users reported chiropractic helping a great deal with their health problem and improving overall health or well-being."[57]

Chiropractic patients were found to be more satisfied with their care after four weeks of treatment than were medical patients. The study also concluded that patients were more satisfied with chiropractic care than they were with physical therapy after six weeks of treatment.[58]

Chiropractic is the largest, most regulated and best recognized of the complementary and alternative medicine (CAM) professions. CAM patient surveys show that chiropractors are used more often than any other alternative provider group and patient satisfaction with chiropractic care is very high. There is steadily increasing patient use of chiropractic in the United States, which has tripled in the past two decades.[59]

In the final analysis, the chiropractic practitioner that can combine his or her extensive skill and training in patient care with the appropriate regimen of therapy is the doctor of choice for today's musculoskeletal pain population. Sound patient coaching, proper exercise and nutritional regimens to strengthen the patient are of great benefit as well while they progress back into an active and enjoyably fit lifestyle.

Why Adjust the Spine?

Hippocrates, the father of modern medicine said, "Look well to the spine for the cause of disease." Socrates, perhaps the greatest philosopher and teacher of all time stated, "If you would seek health, look first to the spine." Modern medicine seems to largely ignore what its practitioners spent long hours in anatomy labs to learn, that the spine and its spinal nerves dictate the function of every organ in our body. Spinal nerves are the vital connection between the brain and its target organs directing the beating of the heart, pumping of the lungs, digesting of our food, hormonal balance of our systems, ovulation, blood flow, male erection and every other bodily function. Many of these functions are thoughtless. We don't have to remember to breathe and those 'involuntary' functions are carried out by our autonomic nervous system a large part or which is carried by our spinal nerves!

Spinal motion is the result of just 24 moving spinal vertebrae that also surround and protect our spinal cords while allowing the exit of our spinal nerves. The spinal nerves, those major lifelines to our organs, exit through small openings known as 'foramen'. Each foramen is formed by the opposing vertebrae. That is to say that the upper half of any foramen is formed by the vertebra above and the lower half by the vertebra below. Unfortunately, 24 movable vertebrae, each side bending, flexing forward and backward and rotating right and left, can slip or shift individually to entrap or compress spinal nerves. These shifts or subluxations can either 'pinch' the nerves directly or produce enough spinal stress to cause swelling of joint tissue adjacent to the nerves. Joint swelling can further compress spinal nerves or produce nerve irritation via inflammation. Either way, the result is an irritated or dysfunctional spinal nerve directing organ function. Subluxations may often cause little pain but the consequences of long-standing nerve compression can be serious. No other condition has so much potential to do us harm. Spinal manipulation lessens compression, stretches adhesions and tight spinal joint capsules while re-establishing spinal mobility and alignment, helping to ensure good nerve flow and neural direction to maintain health and prevent disease.

Keeping our discs healthy and hydrated is another important reason to have your spine adjusted. Unlike most other structures in the human body spinal discs don't have a direct blood supply. Blood flows into the bones of the spine via small blood vessels and then diffuses through the bone and into the discs to provide these important living shock absorbers the nutrients and oxygen they need to replenish, repair and stay healthy.[60] Discs act like sponges for this important exchange and spinal movement is essential to this process. When vertebral motion is lost or altered through abnormal postural stress or mishap vertebral motion can be lost. Without the normal pumping action of a freely moving spine fixed vertebrae do not allow proper diffusion of nutrients into the discs.[61] And so a process of disc starvation begins as discs begin to dry out and the clock on spinal aging starts ticking. The longer the condition remains the more likely that disc damage and degeneration will ensue.

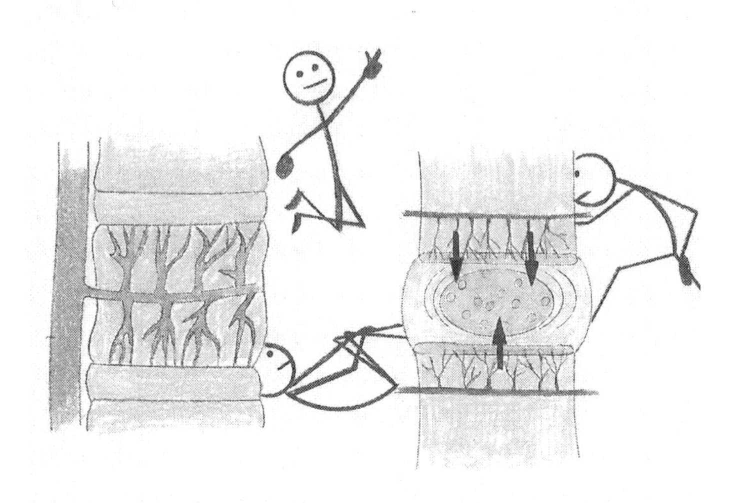

Discs get their blood supply and nutrition when they move freely.

This process also occurs in our spinal joints. Our spine has numerous joints similar to those of our fingers. In fact, a typical single cervical vertebra has a total of eight joints. Animal studies have demonstrated that fixed spinal joints show signs of arthritic change within a matter of weeks.[62]

Spinal manipulation is important, especially with aging. Senior patients who are new to chiropractic care and receive cervical spine manipulation will usually see an immediate improvement in neck movement and balance; a significant boon to daily tasks.

Finally, misaligned spines are either painful now or will be in time. Proper maintenance with good spinal hygiene including posture, exercise and spinal manipulation provides years and years to your health.

A New Specialist Arrives

Today many chiropractors are specializing in fields more formerly thought of as the province of medicine alone. These specialties require several years of advanced training and include radiology, neurology, internal medicine, family practice, pediatrics, sports medicine and in my case orthopedics. For the chiropractor specializing in orthopedics a further three or more years of study and training in the diagnosis and conservative (non-surgical) treatment of muscle, joint and skeletal problems is required. This is followed by extensive clinical and written examinations taking place over two full days or more to receive board certification. Our patient's present with a variety of health problems such as migraine headaches, neck and shoulder pain, disc herniations, sports injuries, low back pain, carpal tunnel pain, sciatica and radiating arm pain, chronic hip/knee/foot or other joint conditions, TMJ disorders and degenerative conditions, etc.. Children are not excluded as we treat various pediatric conditions.

The Chiropractic Orthopedist uses their training to help his or her patients find effective and lasting solutions to ending pain, disability and degenerative changes of the body without surgery or medications. There is no other health care provider who receives such in-depth instruction in non-invasive care for musculoskeletal conditions (MS). Since the Chiropractic Orthopedist does not prescribe medication their success depends on accurately determining the source of a patient's pain and any underlying conditions that are promoting the problem and then dispensing the right therapies and advice to alleviate pain and ensure that timely healing takes place.

For spinal complaints, I recommend seeing either a chiropractor or chiropractic specialist. All have at least four years of graduate-level training and specialists have considerably more. Some of the specialties found among the chiropractic profession include: Chiropractic Radiologist, DACBR, Chiropractic Rehabilitation Specialist, DACRB, Chiropractic Nutritionist, DABCN, Chiropractic Internist, DABCI, Chiropractic Sports Medicine Specialist, DACBSP, Chiropractic Pediatric Specialist, DICCP, Diplomate American Chiropractic Board of Neurology, DACBN, Diplomate American Chiropractic Board of Occupational Health, ACBOH, Diplomate American Board of Chiropractic Acupuncture DABCA and Diplomate American Board of Chiropractic Orthopedists DABCO. For joint conditions, I would make the same recommendation but include the medical orthopedist, medical rheumatologist and podiatrist as primary caregivers.

Final Thoughts

Medical students pledge to follow the Hippocratic Oath, a part of which follows; "I will not be ashamed to say I know not, nor will I fail to call my colleagues when the skills of another are needed for my patient's recovery." While I have great respect for the depth of training and the dedication of medical doctors I am saddened to say that few will admit their limited knowledge of musculoskeletal diagnosis and treatment. It is my hope, that with the passage of time the medical profession will acknowledge the need to refer musculoskeletal patients to a doctor who is better trained to diagnose and treat MS patients. A doctor who uses conservation, cost-effective and non-surgical methods to assist them; a chiropractor.

Healing: Fundamental Concepts

1. Spinal and other forms of bodily pain are usually associated with muscle or soft tissue injury which can, in most cases, heal easily with knowledge and correct practices.

2. We are machines of human design, subject to the same wear and tear as any machine and like any machine, good body alignment is a must. Faulty body mechanics are created by underlying defects such as flat feet, leg length differences, spinal compressions, abnormal spinal curvatures, forward head posture and a host of others that stress our bodies and create pain. To be truly healthy we have to identify these defects and address them.

3. Posture is profound. The postures we employ throughout our working, playing and resting day have a major effect on pain reduction. Correct posture allows our bodies to do what pain medications cannot and that is to heal. Incorrect postures delay healing!

4. The therapy and exercise employed must fit the injury or condition. Using the wrong therapy is guaranteed to keep you in pain!

Charting a Course to Recovery…Where Healing Begins

Finding our way through the maze of treatment options, health care providers, multiple therapies and conflicting opinions can be a confusing and intimidating process. However, recovering from a musculoskeletal condition can be simplified by following the steps below. As you continue to read these steps will be discussed and applied frequently.

Understanding the injury: It's hard to get better if you don't know what's wrong with you! Sounds logical right? Well, you're about to learn that the vast majority of acute and chronic pain is due to soft tissue injuries. Soft tissue injuries are simple to understand and treat. Most spinal conditions can be vastly improved with good spinal care and more serious issues such as rotator cuff tears, knee meniscal injuries, disc herniations and migraine headaches can also be ameliorated without surgery in many cases.

Receiving proper treatment and avoiding harmful therapy: Some therapies heal while other harm. Knowing which therapies are suited for your injury is a must! In the following pages, you'll learn which therapies you require to get better and which ones you should avoid.

Correcting abnormal body mechanics: Human mechanical defects stress our bodies, produce injury and prevent or delay healing. Speedy recovery requires recognition and correct treatment of these varied abnormalities. You'll learn if abnormal mechanics may be affecting you and how best to treat these conditions.

Maintaining good posture: Each painful condition has different postural requirements. We will explore how posture applies to each condition further on.

Performing the right exercises for the condition: Correct exercises performed at the right time and in the right manner, helps heal and strengthen soft tissue injuries. You will learn which are best and which to avoid.

Understanding the nature and timeline of healing and staying the course: Healing takes time. Often weeks or months are needed and some therapies may be necessary long after pain has ended.

As the swelling of damaged tissue reduces from treatment, my patients are dramatically better within a few days or weeks! Feeling great, there are always a few patients who are ready to 'jump ship' and dismiss themselves from care. With a parting goodbye, "Doc I feel great! I don't think I need to come anymore", they are out the door! In spite of my warnings and throwing caution to the wind many quickly forget the advice that got them to their present state! Often these patients return to old habits and within days or weeks are experiencing renewed pain by disregarding those words. Soft tissue healing takes time, good non-stretching posture, proper management and correct therapy to complete the lengthy process of healing and a return to normal physiologic function. There are no shortcuts and no magic bullets.

The Human Machine

The human body is an amazingly complex, self-regulating and healing biological machine possessed of soul, spirit and great intelligence. Our intelligence is often of a kind we cannot see. It is the intelligence of an organism with the complete capacity to maintain itself in perfect health if given pure air, clean water, nourishing food, restorative rest, exercise and peaceful space. Chiropractors call this ability innate; an inner capacity in each of us to heal and restore our bodies and to maintain our health in perfect balance given these proper ingredients. At the heart of this influence is the profound effect of our brain and central nervous system providing the neural nourishment and direction for every bodily organ and tissue. An unfettered and freely functioning nervous system is paramount to the health and sustainability of our human machine.

In my capacity as a chiropractor, I am a healer and a teacher to my patients as I guide them back to health when their human machines have suffered injury or lost balance. I do this in a number of ways: first by educating each patient about the nature of their injury or painful condition and the need for proper rest, posture, exercise, nutrition and other factors necessary for healing. I also ensure that my patients have good nerve flow from their brain and spinal cord to each of their organs via a well-functioning spine, freely moving, without restriction or reduction of their spinal nerve flow with spinal adjustments as needed. But most of all, I help them to understand that they are complete and have a God-given ability to heal and to regulate their own health and well being, as the beneficiaries of having a marvelously complex and self-sustaining human machine.

The Basics of the Spine

The complexity of the human spine cannot be overstated. Imagine a movable column composed of bony segments capable of holding the human skull and brain, while housing, protecting and transmitting our spinal cord and nerves to nourish every organ as it allows us to lift enormous weight. Weight that is then magnified tenfold at the spinal level due to the physics of leverage! Now imagine these tremendous spinal forces at work as we bend, flex, jump and twist with motion.

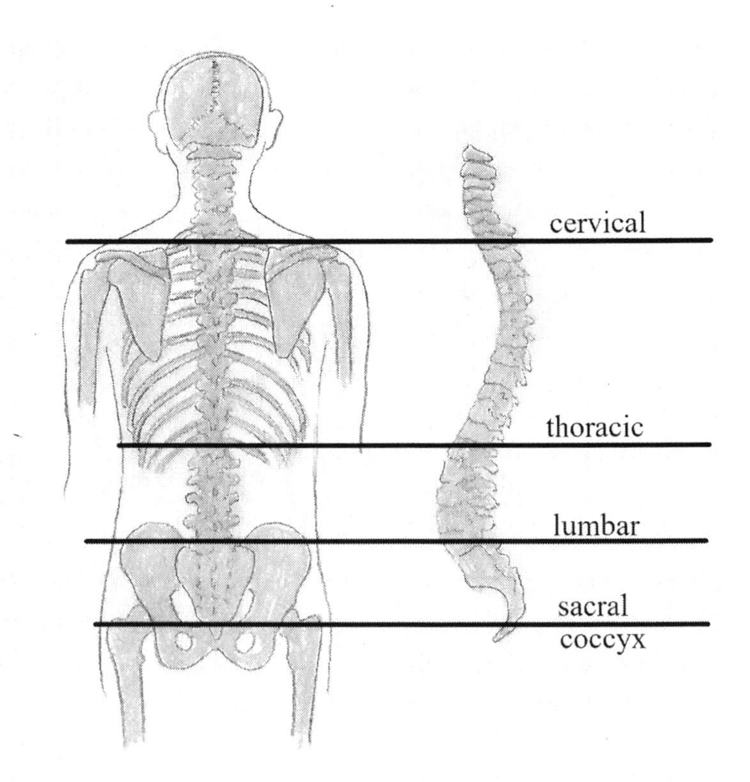

Composed of twenty-four movable vertebrae and two groups of fused vertebrae in the pelvis, the spine begins below the skull and is composed of seven neck or 'cervical vertebrae' normally forming a forward-facing convex curve known as a 'lordotic' curve. This is followed by twelve thoracic vertebrae forming a backward curve known as a 'kyphotic' curve which is in the mid-back between our shoulder blades. These thoracic vertebrae have special 'sockets' for the attachment of our ribs. Next comes five low back or 'lumbar vertebrae' which again form a forward curvature. Finally, at the spine's lowest level we have the sacrum which forms the platform or base for the flexible spine. It is composed of five fused vertebral segments to form a palm-sized bone. The sacrum sits between two large pelvic bones the 'innominates' and shares two large joints with them known as 'sacroiliac joints'. Just below the sacrum is the relatively small coccyx, a collection of three to five often fused vertebrae that form a kind of rudimentary 'tail-like' ending to the spine.

In a perfect world, this would be more than enough to make the human spine complex but we are sometimes imperfect! Imperfection may present in many forms when it comes to spinal architecture. Individual spinal vertebrae are not always uniform in shape. Having multiple growth centers each vertebra may be inadequately formed due to abnormal growth center development producing misshapen vertebra affecting the balance of the vertebrae above as well as altering spinal motion. Further, since in childhood the spine is soft and with much cartilage mishaps and injuries can damage the growth centers as well. Unequal leg length or a deformed pelvis can further this complexity. Adding to the mix, various injuries we incur as adults can produce slippages and off-centering of spinal vertebrae and impair spinal motion, thus creating localized pain and inflammation of spinal components and nerve tissue.

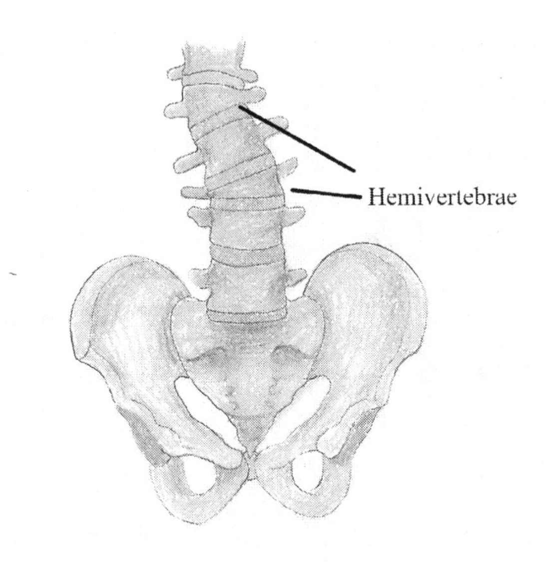

As a result of these imperfections, spinal nerve compression is common and often undiagnosed with unfortunate consequences for the function of the target organs they supply. There is a reason that chiropractors spend four years studying the spine, its complexities and its profound effect on the orchestration of our bodies. No other system is so important to our health. The in-depth training chiropractors receive, in being able to recognize subtle spinal abnormalities is key to solving spinal pain. This coupled with the years of careful practice in the manual manipulation of spinal vertebrae to re-establish good spinal alignment and mechanics makes them far superior to any other health practitioner in the conservative treatment of spinal disorders. Medical radiologists, physical therapists and medical doctors do not have such training and their understanding of these issues is seldom complete. This lack of knowledge can lead to their poor and inconsistent results in treating spinal pain patients.

Spinal Balance

When I think of spinal balance the statuesque posture of the gymnast comes to mind; body erect with the head carried directly over and aligned with the squared shoulder; this line falling straight downward through the hip, knee and ankle. The type of easy and natural balance that brings beauty to form and the symmetry, grace and power to perform the vaults, tumbles and aerial maneuvers required of the gymnast's sport. As a chiropractor, I also think of the natural and normal forward curvatures of the spinal vertebrae in the neck and lower back counterbalanced by the backward curve of the mid-back and pelvis. These are balanced curvatures that allow for a sinuous and rhythmic movement of the spine whenever we walk or run. Movement that allows for the free flow of spinal fluid passing from the brain, downward and surrounding our spinal cord and nerves to nourish them as they control all our bodily functions. This pumping action returns the spinal fluid to the brain in a never-ending cycle.

Unfortunately, a gymnast's posture is more idyllic than real as our lifestyle of over-consumption, over-work and poor sleep habits undermine balance, Spinal defects, both inherited and acquired also take their toll. Looking at a photo of a sunny ocean boardwalk from my grandfather's time it is hard to spot an obese person. Today it's almost as hard to find adults that are fit and trim. Years ago we didn't work or study for hours each day bent over a computer. Postures of daily living, work and sleep, lack of exercise and deconditioning, excess weight or outright obesity, all work against spinal balance. These create the subtle, usually unrecognized body stressors that can damage soft tissue, wear and subluxate (misalign) our spines and lead to chronic pain.

Muscle and the Human Machine

The human body is composed of many types of soft tissue structures that knit our bodies together, muscle by far being the most abundant. Composing over 40% to 45% of our lean body mass our 640 skeletal muscles are covered by thin glistening sheets of fascia. Fascia forms thin membranes to cover and connect individual and adjacent muscles. Toward the ends of muscle, the fascia combines to form rope-like tendons that travel from the ends of the muscles to attach them to bone. Ligaments, another type of soft tissue, bind adjacent bones together expanding at bone endings to form the capsules around our joints. Inside the joints, the surfaces of the meshing bones are surfaced with tough cartilage. Cartilage allows for smooth movement of the joint surfaces as it receives lubricating fluid from 'synovial' tissues lining the non-weight bearing inner walls of the joint capsules. In addition to the cartilage of joints, (such as our fingers, knees or shoulders), special cartilage pads between the vertebrae of the spine called discs, provide movement and shock absorption. Like complex machines, our human muscular motors, ligamentous pulleys, bony levers, meshing joints and shock-absorbing discs and cartilage synchronize to provide graceful movement and power.

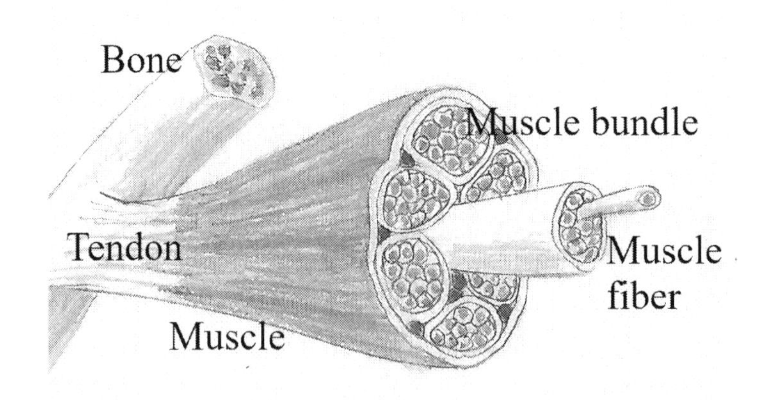

A single muscle, like all soft tissue; discs, tendons, ligaments, etc., is composed of thousands of fibers. These fibers in the muscle are interwoven like the fingers of two hands interlaced. The interwoven fibers slide along each other while maintaining strong cross-links. Muscle fibers roll apart to reach their maximum length during a deep stretch. A hard muscle contraction is achieved by an inward rolling of the fibers to their shortest length, similar to collapsing an extension ladder.

When we contract a muscle, the force generated is dictated by the number of fibers within the muscle working at any one time. We may contract all the fibers at once or only a portion of the fibers depending on our needs. It is the amount of nerve signal flowing from the spinal nerves that determine this response. A little nerve flow produces a slight contraction of a few fibers and we lift a pen. A huge outburst of nerve force and we lift a fallen comrade at arms.

Even One Movement is Complex!

Skeletal muscle moves us by contracting and shortening certain muscle groups while other muscles stabilize such motions as they 'brake' or slow that motion by contracting even as they lengthen. Thus to lift a coffee cup to our lips we must contract the biceps muscle in the front of our arm while lengthening and slightly contracting the triceps muscle in the back of our arm. So it goes, on and on, with every movement of our bodies; some muscles shorten, others lengthen and often the same muscles must do both at some point within the movement!

Complex motions often require hundreds of muscles interacting with precision and skill: a golfer's 'drive', a pitcher's 'curve' ball, the tennis 'slice', all working in synchrony applying just the right amount of force and counterforce needed for the skills required. Human motion is equivalent to a complex orchestral arrangement of musicians providing just the right amplitude of power, tone and integrated timing of a Carnegie Hall performance wherein the conductor is the freely flowing nerve signals coming from brain to spine to muscle.

Complex movements bring about complex forces that can, when extreme or out of balance, damage muscle and other forms of soft 'connective' tissues.

Macro Trauma vs. Micro Trauma

When we think of injury we usually think of something spectacular, a fall or car wreck. Certainly, these can do plenty of damage and such injuries result in 'macro' (major) trauma. But consider the 'daily grind' of the person who sits bending their 12-pound head over a keyboard or pitched forward to see a cell phone or computer screen. Consider the commuter in stressful positions of sitting as they bounce or jar their way to and from work, or the damage done in stomach sleeping as we twist our neck for hours placing stress on delicate spinal joints night after night. Soon these postures bring painful burning in the neck or back and perhaps the onset of headaches. This we call subtle or 'microtrauma'. Microtrauma can slowly degrade the connective tissues of muscle, tendon, ligament and cartilage leading to chronic pain and degenerative changes in these tissues and their joints.

Microtrauma also results from the wear and tear our bodies experience when we are out of balance! Like any machine, we can wear out. This is especially true when one or more structural defects stress our bodies! Over the years I have looked at many hip x-rays. The largest single reason for severe hip degeneration and arthritis is a difference in leg length! Leg length differences are common and yet seldom mentioned in radiology reports. The consequences of leg length inequality are immense. Moving on legs of different lengths stresses the low back, hip sockets, knees and ankles. Over time cartilage in the affected joints is eroded and when thin enough, arthritic changes appear. I often explain it to patients this way: imagine operating your car with 15-inch tires on one side of the vehicle and 16-inch tires on the other side; do you think you might have some knocks, squeaks and rattles after a while?

How Muscles Tear and Heal

Muscle is designed to contract but muscle and other forms of soft tissue can only stretch so far! When a muscle is stretched past its breaking point, individual muscle fibers begin to tear and this we term muscle 'strain'.[63] Typically, only a very small percentage of these fibers are damaged and often in a diffuse or spread-out fashion. As a result, the vast majority of the muscle fibers remain intact and therefore still strong and capable of function. However, the tissue damage and the resulting inflammatory response can be extremely painful. Swelling may take several hours to develop with increasingly severe pain confusing the victim as they may remember no trauma. Severe pain may result and I have literally seen grown men and women, (and by the way, the women are usually tougher), assisted into my office unable to stand due to the severe pain and weakness of muscle injuries. This is not so hard to understand when one considers that in addition to the increased pressure inside the damaged muscle from excess swelling, various inflammatory chemicals are released from damaged muscle fibers chemically irritating surrounding pain nerve receptors. Such muscle injuries can be so painful that any movement brings rapid, intense and crippling body pain that we confuse with spasm. As you will soon learn however, muscle spasm is a rarity!

Recognizing Body Imbalance

The human body may be affected by a constellation of faulty body mechanics or 'biomechanical' defects causing injury, pain and wear. If we are to be well and age well these defects need to be identified and corrected if possible. Recognizing these faults, their impact on your health and providing correct treatment is the forte of the chiropractor and the specialty of the chiropractic orthopedist.

Body imbalance has many forms:

- Forward head posture (FHP) when the head is held in front of its normal balance point over the erect shoulder; requiring the muscles of the neck and upper back to constantly strain to hold the head aloft eventually resulting in a host of symptoms like headaches, jaw, neck and upper back pain, TMJ, vertigo and balance issues
- Bowed shoulders: exerting a downward force on the mid-back creating pain and the abnormal forces leading to spinal fracture and the spinal collapse of Dowager's Hump
- Reversed or excessive curves of the neck or lower back: stressing our spinal discs and joints, leading to early spinal

disc degeneration capable of compressing spinal nerves and diminishing their ability to properly innervate our organs
- Differences in leg length (quite common) and pelvis or spine defects: capable of producing scoliosis or chronic spinal pain
- Flat feet and ankle pronation: leading to plantar fasciitis, metatarsalgia (forefoot pain), heel spurs, bunions and knee injuries including torn cartilage and retaining ligaments

All of these topics will be discussed in greater detail later in this book.

The Good News and the Time Line of Healing

The human body has an amazing capacity to heal. Muscle is a prime example. During the first few days following an injury, muscle tissue becomes less swollen if no more irritation or trauma is allowed to occur and a mix of 'glue-like' proteins form a rough or 'randomized' patch at the tear sites. Rather than being replaced in a linear or parallel fashion like normal muscle fibers, the replacement fibers overlap in all directions. These fibers are weak and easily torn again and care must be taken to avoid maneuvers and postures that will overstretch repairing fibers at the injury site. This is the stage that most people relate to as stiffness in the area of injury thinking incorrectly that stretch is needed.

Over many weeks if the wound is left to heal without further stretch or injury the patch gets less randomized and fiber orientation becomes more 'linear' in direction, gradually assuming the appearance and function of strong, healthy muscle tissue. This process is a slow evolution of tissue healing over time and is easily disrupted with strenuous activities, over-stretching, massage and incorrect therapies.[64]

There are three distinct phases of healing and while it is difficult to put a precise time frame on any one of them due to the variety of injury, the condition, age and health of the patient and the therapies utilized, a general model and time-line can be given. Remember however, if you're constantly overworking, over-stretching or doing the wrong therapy you'll stay in the inflammatory phase...forever!

1. The Inflammatory Phase: Initially after injury tissue swells with pain, redness and increased temperature due to blood accumulation and clotting. The swelling and damage to small blood capillaries, (tiny blood vessels), cut off oxygen to the tissues in the damaged area and cells start to die. Our bodies then produce cells to invade the area to digest the debris. This process normally takes up to three weeks but varies greatly on the degree of tissue damage and blends into phase two.
2. Regeneration and Repair Phase: After the first few days and up to six weeks the body starts to regenerate tissue as fibroblasts begin to lay down collagen (protein) repair fibers to form a randomly oriented fiber patch as new capillaries grow into the area of the damaged area.
3. Remodeling Phase: Over the next few weeks to months the body is fine-tuning the repair and reorganizing the weak and randomly oriented patch laid down in the regeneration phase. With time and proper therapy, the fibers in the damaged area become increasingly aligned with the normal non-damaged muscle fibers surrounding them as they become stronger. During this time they are also becoming more physiologically normal and better at functioning as a contractile unit.

While nearly everyone equates the absence of pain with complete healing and wellness this is a big mistake! Soft tissue inflammation produces swelling, creates pain and is directly proportional to it! Tissue inflammation and pain depart early in the process of healing and well before the injury has resolved. The very delicate and randomized tissue patch or intramuscular 'scab' is just beginning to change its structure toward more normal tissue when swelling and pain have dissipated. Mistaking the absence of pain as a sign of complete healing of a muscle or other soft tissue tear and resuming activity too early is the greatest reason for re-injury and developing chronic pain.

Learning to Heal

The majority of new patients I have seen over these past many years have experienced muscle and other forms of soft tissue injuries . Through bad advice or bad instincts, they massage, poke, prod, vibrate and stretch their damaged muscles, ligaments, tendons and joints keeping them in pain. They often couple this with the wrong therapy and the most damaging, sloppy postures guaranteed to ensure they never get better. While many have spinal issues as well, it is vitally important to know how to heal damaged soft tissue. Now that we know how muscle and other soft tissue are damaged let's find how to heal them.

The Myth of Stretching

Over the years I've worked with many thousands of pain sufferers. Almost to a man or woman when describing back or neck pain, the term they use the most is spasm. Seldom seen in clinical practice, patients typically use the word spasm to describe the stiffness and swelling pressure associated with muscle injuries. Inflammation creates swelling and swelling feels tight which patients mistake for spasm especially when movements may bring on sudden severe pain and a reflexive but momentary 'clinching' contraction of damaged muscles when used!

The times I have taken a case history while a patient describes their neck, elbow, shoulder or leg pain as they constantly kneed, goad or rub the painful area have been too numerous to count. Other images come to mind: the woman describing her chronic right-sided low back pain while crossing her right leg over the left leg she bends forward in her seat (stretching her lower back muscles) as she explains to me her long weeks of pain. Or the tearful young basketball star, as he stretches his left arm behind him while telling me of the left shoulder pain that has benched him in his final season.

Admittedly, stretching brings temporary relief from pain. Stretch, massage and movement messages are carried by receptor nerves that are well insulated by fatty membranes allowing for their fast transmission to our spine and brain. This allows us to have immediate knowledge about the position, pressure and tension on our body parts; information we dearly need to avoid further injury to our bodies! However, pain nerves have little to no fatty coverings and therefore pain information travels much slower from damaged tissue to our spine and brain. Thus our brain gives precedence to messages about stretch, position, pressure and joint tension as it largely ignores pain signals! Pain signals are also blocked at the spinal level as faster signals are quickly routed through!

Many people feel little pain while moving because of this selective scrutiny. However, pain often returns with a vengeance when movement stops! Stretch and massage also increase blood flow, temporarily warming our damaged tissues but there is a cost involved. Each cycle of stretch or massage continues to damage soft tissue injuries prolonging pain while delaying healing. Thus a brief respite from pain during and following stretching quickly passes as pain soon returns with renewed swelling at the injury site.

So let's imagine a superficial cut whose scab is forming in the initial phases of healing. Tearing away the scab can delay healing indefinitely and lead to pronounced scarring at the site. Similarly, deep stretching, massage, vibration, vigorous exercises or overly forceful spinal manipulation of the damaged area can all disrupt, delay and prevent healing by constantly tearing away the internal repairs your body is attempting to make! In separate studies conducted in 1995 and 1997, massage (which mechanically damages healing soft tissue and is another form of stretch) was not shown to be an effective treatment modality for reducing muscle damage after injury or enhancing long term restoration of post-exercise muscle strength.[65,66]

We are lucky that soft tissue strains (usually muscle fiber tears) are not exposed to air thus oxidizing and scaring as readily as are superficial cuts to our skin. However muscle and other soft tissue injuries require much longer to heal than superficial wounds and therefore great care must be taken to keep an injured body part in a neutral position, non-stressed and non-stretched!

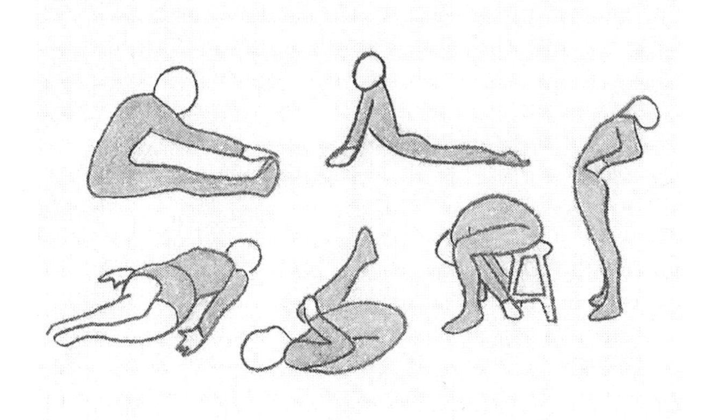

Stretches to avoid with
soft tissue injuries

No single activity is more damaging to torn muscle than stretching! While stretching provides temporary pain relief it does so at the expense of damaging tissues engaged in the slow process of healing. Healing takes weeks and often months. Stretching fragile tissues is akin to tearing the scab off a wound! Improper therapies like stretch, massage, vibration and trigger-point therapy combined with sloppy posture halt soft tissue healing.

Spasm or Muscle Strain?...The 'Hargis Sway Test'

In a perfect world, it would be great to have an easy way to identify spasm and there is! For some years now I've been using a simple test I developed to help me identify the presence of spasm in my patients. I call this maneuver the 'Hargis Sway Test'. For the mid and lower back, you simply have the patient stand with his or her back to you and observe the motion created when you grasp both hips and rotate them gently back and forth. The forward and backward motion created when you rock one hip forward in advance of the other and repeat rhythmically imparts a gentle swaying to the torso that cannot be performed if the back is in spasm. If the lower back and torso move freely and yet the patient has back pain then a soft tissue strain is highly likely!

For the neck, you simply grasp the shoulders standing behind the patent and ask them to fix their gaze upon a forward object and maintain that gaze while you rotate the shoulders back and forth with sufficient movement to alter the course of their gaze. If the head stays centered and gaze can be maintained on the object before them then again there is no spasm. In this case spasm of the upper back and neck would prevent the head's rotation to maintain its easy and forward centered gaze. Alternately one can rapidly rock the shoulders noting a gentle neck sway similar to that of the lower back. Why do I mention the test? Because adopting this test alone would simplify the diagnosis of back pain and save substantial amounts of money, time and suffering! Do it at home and satisfy yourself that spasm is likely not a component of your problem.

Visit HealingTheHumanMachine.com for a video of the 'Hargis Sway Test'.

Chances are you are one of the nine out of ten pain sufferers that do not have spasm but are usually incorrectly treated as if you did with stretch, massage, vibration and overly forceful exercise.

A Simple Little Test for Muscle Damage

Since our bodies have a lot of muscle, (even under the fat), it isn't hard to find them. When you have pain in the neck, shoulder, low back, hip, buttock, leg, etc., you can 'palpate' the area of pain to test for muscular injury. Just press into the areas of muscular tissue with moderate to deep finger pressure. For neck and low back pain press one to two inches lateral to or away from the spine. If you have buttock pain press into the buttock muscles themselves. If your experiencing mid-back pain press into the muscle and tendon area just inside the shoulder blades. For leg pain probe the posterior or lateral leg and calf. If moderate to deeper finger pressure produces pain and yet you can move the area (even with some pain on movement) you likely have soft tissue damage and no spasm.

(Deep leg pain particularly in the posterior calf, can indicate a blood clot or deep vein thrombosis DVT. This is fairly uncommon but can be quite serious. Blood clots are usually associated with swelling, pain, tenderness, increased warmth of the area and often a pale, bluish or red discoloration. The American Society of Hematology estimates that a DVT affects as many as 900,000 Americans each year. One hundred thousand Americans die annually from complications related to this disorder, particularly when a blood clot breaks free of its vascular origin usually in an extremity and travels to the heart, lungs or brain. If you have severe deep pain or pain primarily in an extremity associated with the above signs you should seek emergency medical care immediately.)

When is Muscle Spasm Likely?

Muscle spasm is uncommon but does occur. Any acute slippage of a vertebra is capable of pinching a spinal nerve with near-instant spasm. Alternately spinal fracture, especially with bony displacement, may engender spasm. The major and defining difference between true spasm and the severe momentary or 'clinching' pain related to a strained muscle is the duration of muscle seizure. Spasms don't let up and may be sustained for minutes or hours. Pain from a muscle strain however, is momentary, coming in waves with movement or position changes and then just as quickly subsiding when muscular stress is diminished. Figuring out the difference is critical because proper care for each varies widely. Muscle strains need rest, ice, ultrasound, no stretch and healing. Spasm needs stretch, heat and movement. So let's look at a few instances when spasm may occur.

A lumbar disc herniation may cause spasm in the form of an involuntary sidewards or forwards tilt of the torso. Health professionals' term this 'antalgia' and basically, it is the body's way of reducing spinal cord or nerve pressure by pulling the spine into a position of less compression. If you find yourself with acute back pain, (and in many cases leg pain and numbness often traveling to the foot), with an inability to straighten your torso, there is a better than even chance that you are experiencing antalgia due to acute 'partial' disc tear or true herniation. Most often this tilting of the torso will subside within a few days if managed properly and usually does not require surgery but may respond beautifully to bed rest in a supine position with one pillow under the head and another under the knees, ice packs and ultrasound. If leg pain and numbness are present spinal traction may be indicated as well. (Spinal traction, which is highly effective in reducing spinal disc herniations, will be discussed later on.)

Similarly, very rapid onset of mid-back pain, with an inability to take a deep breath due to limited chest expansion, is a strong signal that you have slippage of a spinal vertebra or rib head with spasm as a component. Spinal slippage requires spinal manipulation which is very effective in quickly reducing pain and restoring proper spinal or rib placement. These instances are much less common than strain, sprain or soft tissue injury.

In this day of fast food, the poor nutritive value of foods grown on depleted soil and abusive lifestyles with overconsumption of diuretics such as coffee and alcohol, we tend to have less mineral intake than we require and often retain less as well. This can lead to restless leg syndrome and leg cramps. Supplementation with a good multi-mineral source combining calcium, potassium and magnesium is usually the key to resolving such issues by restoring blood mineral balance.

Finally, prolonged stress to a body part mechanically overloaded and imbalanced can result in increased tension in muscle structures. This is often seen in forward head displacement or when the pelvis is not level due to and leg length inequalities. Most commonly nodular spasms or 'knots' will occur within the structure of individual muscles. These focal areas of spasm are often termed 'trigger points' and can respond to therapy of the same name. Mainly this entails holding a deep sustained pressure to the area to 'release' the contraction. This is risky however since most tight muscles are more often the result of swelling secondary to acute strain.

Determining the difference between spasm and strain should be less confusing now that you know how to 'palpate' for tenderness and to use the 'Sway Test'.

Gait Related Leg Pain vs. Sciatica

Almost everyone with leg pain tells me they have sciatica but true sciatic leg pain is uncommon. There's an old song that goes, "The foot bone's connected to the leg bone, the leg bone's connected to the knee bone, the knee bone's connected to the thigh bone, etc., you get my drift. The foot, ankle, knee, lower and upper leg, hip and lower back are all part of a 'movement chain'. Have you ever noticed how people with back, hip or leg pain limp? How they alter their gait to get on and off the painful leg/hip quickly in an attempt to lessen their pain? Often back or hip pain sufferers will also 'sway' side to side, as they move with their pain. Any injury to these areas may cause us to walk or move in patterns differing from our norm. Within a few days, the muscles of the back and leg stressed by an abnormal gait will become tender confusing the patient who imagines they are developing sciatica. Health providers poorly trained will usually assume the same! This can lead to a host of unnecessary tests and treatment.

Secondary leg strain from limping presents as a classical pattern; pain is located in the lateral or posterior buttock, lateral hip or leg to the lateral knee often extending down into the lateral side of the calf but seldom to the foot. Such pain presents as a diffuse (ill-defined and spread out) soreness without numbness. Direct pressure into the painful regions will reproduce pain in the strained muscular regions. The bottom line: don't limp. A more normal and smooth transition from foot to foot during walking will require more duration on the painful side but will pay huge dividends in lessening pain and faster healing! Take it easy with a smooth steady gait.

True sciatic pain is usually due to a slipped or shifted spinal vertebrae and/or disc injury with nerve compression. A disc that has herniated to the left will often cause left leg pain extending in a direct line to and including the foot with a hot electric wire sensation, shocking, buzzing, sharp or dull and is often accompanied by numbness of the lower leg or foot. Often there is an associated weakness of the foot or leg as well. Deep tendon reflexes may be slowed or absent in addition producing a reduced 'patellar' jerk reflex below the knee or a diminished Achilles tendon reflex at the rearward ankle. Bowel or bladder function may be affected as well. Confusing even to most health practitioners, my recommendation is to always consult the most learned practitioner one can find to sort these symptoms out!

Visit HealingTheHumanMachine.com for a video discussing secondary leg strain and sciatica.

Any low back, hip, leg, knee or foot pain can alter the way we walk resulting in limping or other abnormal patterns of movement straining the muscles of the leg. Secondary leg strain represents the most common reason for leg pain and is far more common than sciatica.

Regional Injury and Pain Migration

Many of my patients show great concern when in the midst of treatment their pain seems to shift in location. However, it's rare to injure just one muscle or soft tissue component. Most muscle strains are regional, affecting several contiguous muscle groups, some more severely damaged than others. Secondary muscle strain will also occur to other areas of a movement chain as discussed previously. Initially, therapy is directed to the most painful areas. As more severely injured soft tissues improve other areas of strain may arise as primary complaints since our brain tends to focus on the area of greatest pain intensity to the seeming extinction of lesser pain sites! With proper therapy and healing, the area most painful initially, will improve and other regions of damage may become more noticeable.

In more complex cases when there may be true spinal pain due to disc injury, spinal joint inflammation or vertebral misalignment coupled with muscle injury, whichever is the more dominant in terms of pain intensity may improve resulting in pain moving to the lesser source. Pain may begin centrally in the spine and then seem to move laterally into the flank, buttock, hip or leg or vice versa. In these cases all areas are pain productive but not to the same degree and so with greater healing in some areas pain again will alter in location.

How to Sit for Low Back Pain...Avoiding Slumpville

How we sit is so important to the course of low back pain that it deserves its own section. Whenever I see a new low back patient you can be sure this is a conversation we're having on day one! Since the vast majority of low back pain includes some degree of muscle injury, sitting without stretching the lumbar muscles is essential for healing. Unfortunately, most of us sit either slumped or leaning forward toward a computer screen. Seated postures that resemble a 'cheese curl', stretch muscle and other soft tissues in the back and pelvis and is a leading player in chronic back pain. Computer sitting, as we lean forward or downward toward computer monitors, sitting in bed with pillows propping you up or sitting on very low chairs, low bleachers, the floor or a low toilet stool, promote over-stretching of the lower back and will prolong and intensify low back pain, sciatica and disc pathology. A good rule to remember is to never sit so low as to have your knees higher than your hips while sitting; if you do you are sitting slumped!

Another big culprit, especially in the American household, is the couch; typically, soft and non-supportive, allowing our backs to bow rearward into 'slumpville'. This is compounded when we place our feet up on a hassock or coffee table forming a 90 degree or L shape between our torso, back and elevated legs creating a subtle ongoing stretch over minutes or hours. Many patients remark on near-crippling back pain when they try to arise and straighten from this position! Placing pillows behind the back, while continuing to sit on a soft couch, is rarely beneficial.

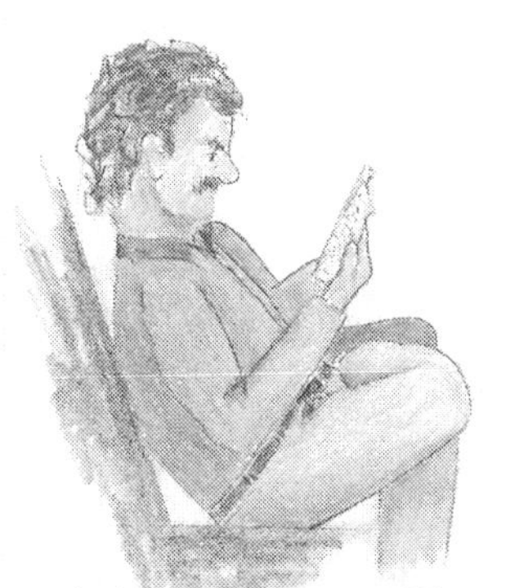

Sitting in 'slumpville' overstretching the back, buttock, hip and leg

How to sit? Textbooks will tell you to sit erect in a supportive chair with your feet on the floor. This is fine for general applications and in the work environment, a full back office chair with forward lumbar support is a plus. Office chairs with the typical oval support for the mid and upper back with nothing at all for the lower back should be avoided. At home, my pick for the best seating is the recliner. A good recliner should offer firm support for the lower back and allow the user to move their lower back firmly against the back support and then allow for a reclining position with feet and legs elevated. This position has the advantage of allowing the user to lean backward before elevating the legs which 'opens up' the lower back allowing a much wider angle between the torso and lower extremities, than that obtained while sitting on a couch and using a hassock. This wider angle reduces stretch/stress to the lower back and is a fine way to rest while slipping an appropriately covered ice pack behind the back for 15 minutes each hour to allow for a comfortable way to reduce swelling associated with back pain.

This position can also be adapted to driving and I encourage my low back pain patients to elevate their car seat beneath them so that the seat is raised to make it flatter and more bench-like. Following this, I advise reclining the backrest to again open up the angle of the lower back to more than 90 degrees. This position when coupled with lumbar support found in most vehicles provides a less stressful position while driving. If you have no lumbar support in your vehicle you can buy an after-market support or improvise with a bit of foam or a small folded towel.

Visit HealingTheHumanMachine.com for a brief video on sitting positions.

Sleep Position Can Make or Break Your Pain

The shortest distance between two points is a straight line. When we stand effect, sit erect and lie straight on our backs we are allowing our bodies to be in a more relaxed and less stressed position. Sleep and sitting positions are vitally important to heal soft tissue injuries but this is a discussion few pain sufferers ever have with their doctor. So a few simple rules should be followed to get the best healing and restorative sleep! If you have...

- Back, hip or buttock pain on both sides; sleep on the back with one small pillow beneath the head and one beneath the knees.
- Back, hip or buttock pain on only one side; sleep on the back or with the painful side upward with a long pillow between the legs. This allows the upper leg of the painful side to stay elevated preventing the inner knee of the upper leg to come down and rest on the mattress, (a position to avoid as it is capable of stretching the back, buttock, hip and lateral leg on the painful side).

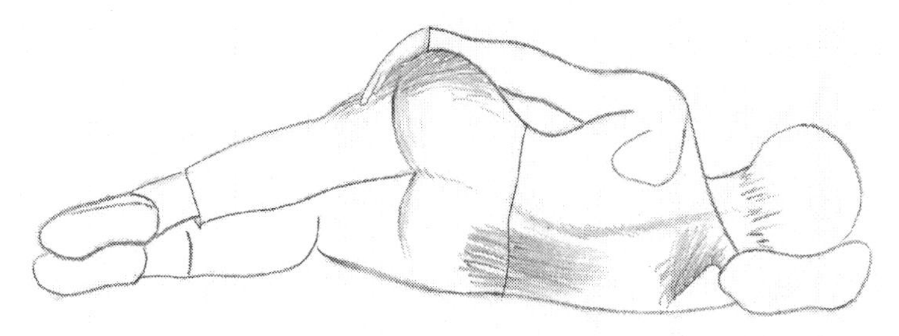

Side sleeping can overstretch muscles in the shoulder, low back, hip and buttock.

- One-sided or bilateral mid back pain requires the same positions as those listed above for the low back.
- Knee pain; sleep on the back with a pillow under the painful knee or on your side with the painful knee uppermost and on top of a long pillow placed between the knees; preventing the 'bad' knee to rest on the mattress. (Resting the upper painful knee on the mattress stretches the inner components of the knee.)
- Shoulder pain; sleep on the non-painful side or back with the arm of the painful shoulder always down and never over the head or under the pillow. (Both positions impinge shoulder structures including the rotator cuff tendons. Avoiding overhead arm positions, is especially important for those with biceps tendon instability as in this position the long head of the biceps tendon tends to slip out of its normal position in the bicipital groove increasing instability.) Simultaneous right and left shoulder pain require sleeping on one's back. Often hugging a pillow to the chest is helpful.
- Pain inside the shoulder blade on one side; sleep on your back or with the painful side up if side sleeping. Bilateral shoulder blade pain requires sleeping on the back only. The arm on the painful side should always be down.
- Neck pain on one side; sleep with the painful side upward,

your head slightly elevated toward the upper shoulder.

- Neck pain on both sides; sleep on the back with a small to medium-sized pillow.
- Carpal Tunnel, Wrist, Elbow, Arm Pain; sleep on your side with the painful side upward or on your back. Never place your carpal tunnel hand under your pillow as the weight of your head atop the pillow will transfer pressure to the carpal area. Lastly, never flex the wrist to rest the palm or backside of your carpal tunnel hand on the mattress, as these positions reduce the carpal space compressing nerve structures.
- Multiple Areas of Pain; back sleeping is a must for it is in this position that none of our body parts are stretched or stressed. A small to medium pillow placed under the head and knees compliments this position.

Visit HealingTheHumanMachine.com for a brief video on sleep positions.

Back sleep allows all our body parts to be linear and our tissues to rest in a non-stretched fashion. This position is also restorative to tissue injuries, giving minor strains that we may experience during our daily work or play a chance to heal. (Back sleeping is especially good for amateur and professional athletes to allow optimal healing between engagements.)

Patients will sometimes complain of slow results during treatment. Questioning them further, they usually admit to a lapse in the recommended postures sometimes for just a few minutes. As we have learned injured muscle fibers are delicate threads seeking to reunite and heal. Bad postures stretch these healing threads. How long does it take to break a thread? Bottom line; at no time should posture lapse.

Crafting Can Hurt You

As you will learn in the pages to come, forward head posture (FHP) is a leading cause of neck and upper back pain. FHP greatly increases the work your muscles have to do to keep your head erect; crafting with the head flexed downward increases these forces even more. If you're experiencing acute of chronic neck pain try to minimize these activities while proper therapy reduces your pain. If your work involves neck flexion try to elevate monitors, use standing desks, change glasses, use paper holders on the side of computer monitors or in short do anything to reduce head flexion. The same rule applies to cradling phones; get a headset.

Muscle Injuries Will Make You Wake Up Stiff and Sore

The first thing most people with muscular injuries do on arising is stretch due to the profound stiffness/soreness they experience as a result of the muscle healing taking place! Did I say healing? You bet. When muscles have been strained they heal by laying down protein glues, (I'm keeping it simple here), to reconnect and restructure the damaged muscle fibers. Probably no single act is more damaging to the healing process than stretching or massaging painful muscle tissue, especially on waking! This disrupts an entire night during which the body is attempting to form a scab or rough patch as it begins the long process of healing damaged muscle or other forms of soft tissue!

Hopefully, you've slept in a position conducive to healing, (see postures that heal) and your body is doing its job of repairing the damaged soft tissue by laying down what amounts to an internal scab. Stretching at this time (or at any time during the early and mid phases of healing) will re-tear damaged tissue and disrupt the healing process effectively winding back the clock on healing and ensuring renewed and increased levels of pain!

What to do upon arising? Definitely, do not set on the edge of the bed and reach down to the floor to pick up socks. (Too much stretching!) Move gingerly out of bed and walk as smoothly as possible, gently transitioning your weight from leg to leg, without limping. If sitting, sit upright and have a warm but not extremely hot shower, avoiding the tub especially if you have spinal pain in the neck or back as tub contours are likely to allow slumping and stretch to healing tissues. Warm-up slowly and you're off to a good start!

Grading Your Pain… the Analog Scale

Clinicians and patients need an easy way to rate pain and the analog pain scale does just that. Think of the worse pain possible and rate that pain as a ten and the absence of pain a zero. On the analog scale, moderate pain might be a 4 or 5 and more severe pain a 7 or 8. This scale is useful as it provides a practical method of expressing our pain. We know how we felt last week and therefore in a simple number system, we can update ourselves or our health providers. For children too young to use the analog scale numerically, there is a visual scale of faces from very happy to very sad they can point to reflecting their level of discomfort. Numerous examples may be found online.

Ultrasound; Healing Deeply with Acoustic Streaming

My number one therapy for soft tissue healing these past three decades has been ultrasound. Therapeutic ultrasound as a treatment modality has been used by therapists for the last 60 years. Like diagnostic ultrasound, therapeutic ultrasound can penetrate deeply through tissues. Ultrasonic waves, (sound waves of a very high frequency, 800,000 to 2,000,000 cycles per second, are produced by the ultrasound applicator head as it is moved over the surface of the body. A special ultrasound gel is placed on the skin to effectively convey the sound waves into the body. For irregular surfaces like the hand or foot, the applicator and body part can be placed in a water bath during treatment. A 2002 study by J.L. Kames and H.W. Burton in the Archives of Physical Medicine and Rehabilitation demonstrated that seven days of consecutive ultrasound treatment produced significant healing and a return of strength to damaged muscle tissue.[67]

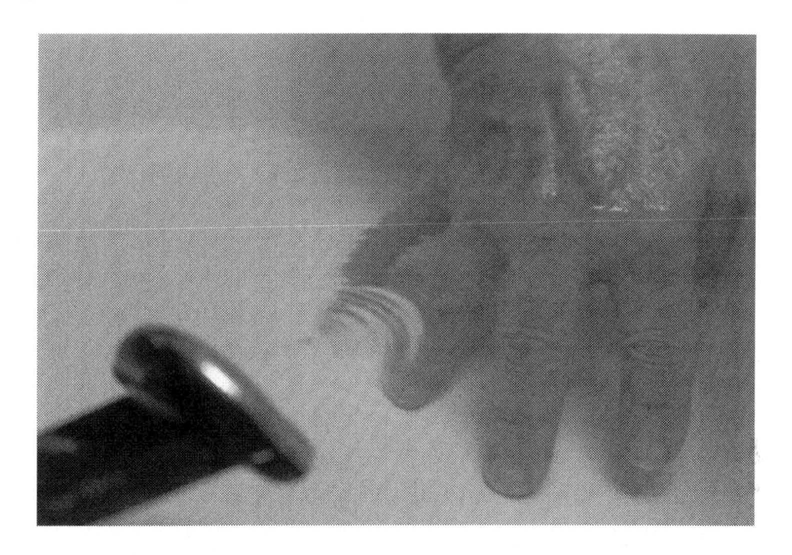

Therapeutic ultrasound works by producing acoustic streaming. Acoustic streaming is best understood when the ultrasound applicator is placed in water. The sound waves produced push the water forward in a rippling or fountain effect! Unfortunately, badly damaged soft tissue areas may be so swollen that the turgid, high-pressure injury region limits the exchange of fluids, healing proteins and other cellular components. Ultrasound accelerates wound healing and tissue repair by reducing stagnant high-pressure swelling in the area of injury, increasing blood flow and stimulating the production of new tissue. Ultrasound also promotes remodeling of damaged tissue and the softening and resolution of scar tissue which may have formed after months or years of chronic injury! (Ultrasound is a medical device and should only be used by a licensed professional health care provider. A therapeutic, professional class ultrasound unit costs about $2000.00 dollars and cheaper units commonly advertised seldom or never compare.)

Ultrasound is truly an amazing therapy and when coupled with good ergonomics, ice packs, good nutrition, mild therapeutic exercise, supplements, rest and cessation of tissue disruptors, (like stretch, massage, vibration and excessive exercise), allows the body to heal! Ultrasound is a mainstay therapy of many chiropractic and physical therapy offices.

Ice is Nice

Home therapy can make or break our efforts to heal and of great importance is icing soft tissue injuries at the correct times. Ice or cold pack applications reduce swelling by producing an initial narrowing of blood vessels called vasoconstriction. After a few minutes of icing an increase of blood vessel width (vasodilation) allows more blood flow to the small blood vessels known as capillaries. This reduces swelling, cleans out damaged cellular debris and promotes healing. Cold applications reduce pain by blocking painful nerve messages both at the tissue and spinal cord levels as it reduces the velocity and intensity of pain nerve transmission. Many incorrectly advise the use of ice packs for only the first 48 hours following an injury but when swelling is prolonged or severe does this apply? Certainly not! As we have seen, pain and swelling can be chronic and cold is beneficial when tissue injury and inflammation is ongoing and unresolved.

Cold can be applied as often as once per hour for up to 15 minutes by placing a moldable gel-type cold pack, atop a lightly misted or moistened towel and then onto the painful body part. As a general rule, I instruct my patients to continue ice pack application at any pain level above a 2. A pain level of 2-4 may allow for a lessening of applications but icing should be continued at least a couple of times per day in my opinion. A pain level of 5 or more is best managed by hourly applications of ice if practical.

Normally ice is safe to use for all injuries but a few contraindications must be observed and would include impaired circulation as in Raynaud's Disease, peripheral vascular disease or insufficiency, (a tendency for blood clots in the extremities), hypersensitivity to cold or skin desensitization, open wounds or skin disorders and infections. (Using ice or cold packs for more than 15 minutes or with too wet a towel can freeze and damage tissue and should be avoided!)

Shoes Too!

Two years before seeing me, Tiffany, a new patient, had been told she needed a total knee replacement. She had punished her knees as a dancer in her younger years and had torn her knee meniscus in a skiing injury. She saw a good surgeon and had an excellent result. Her rehab had been prolonged and very painful and Tiffany was now having lots of problems with the other knee. Dreading a second surgery, Tiffany came to see me. X-rays indicated little cartilage remaining in the right non-operated knee which is never a good sign. On exam, I saw that she was a 'heavy' walker, seeming to 'pound the floor', in place of having a smooth and light step. Examining her shoes and asking about footwear, she gravitated toward leather shoes with little give.

Shoe soles vary greatly; some have soles that are shock absorbing. Both of us having a common day off from work, I traded Tiffany a lunch for meeting her at a large athletic supply store to see if I could find her a more shock-absorbing shoe. After an hour and looking at over a hundred pairs of sports sneakers, testing each sole with my thumb to gage cushioning, I found one that seemed truly exceptional; the New Balance 775.

Tiffany bought a pair and three weeks later she canceled her up-coming surgery. Tiffany had done it all; ultrasound therapy, rehab exercise, listened to my coaching on walking more smoothly, using a pillow between and under her knees in sleeping, avoided placing her feet upon a hassock with her knees hanging unsupported in space and was taking curcumin a natural anti-inflammatory.

Footwear has a huge impact on back and lower extremity pain. There's no doubt that Tiffany got her monies worth when she bought me lunch.

Rehabilitation Exercises: When, Why, How

Soft tissue injuries which again are typically muscular in nature need time to heal. The first stage of healing is at a point when swelling has decreased substantially and a rough patch or primary internal 'scab' has formed. This process typically takes two to six weeks if one is receiving the correct therapies and following the proper postures and habits. (Obviously overworking, long travel, poor posture and incorrect therapy can delay this process indefinitely as previously discussed.) This scab state or 'first intention' healing, (see 'The Time Line of Healing', discussed earlier), also coincides with that point on the analog pain scale when we have lessened our pain to a 1 or 2 in most cases. It is at this time that mild rehab exercises can begin.

Why rehab exercise? Because the right combination of exercise can speed healing, increasing blood flow, oxygenation and nourishment to damaged tissues. Each contraction of healthy muscle fibers assists injured muscle fiber components to reform structurally and physiologically. The only allowable exercises are those of contraction, including both concentric (moving a weight toward our body) and eccentric (moving a weight away from our body), done using very light weights initially or even the weight of only a body part against gravity. Stretch bands offering different levels of resistance can also be used. Absolutely no stretching is to be done during the early phases of exercise.

When is Stretching a Good Thing?

This book is based on my clinical experience and the recognition that most episodes of physical pain are the result of inflammation and damage to tissue. In these cases early stretching in the acute phase prevents healing. However, when healing has reduced the pain completely and a course of rehab strengthening exercise has been underway for several days or even a few weeks mild stretches can begin. These should be done very gently over many days, slowly progressing as we realize that our bodies even with no pain may be healing for several more weeks or months and still somewhat fragile. Unfortunately, there is no good benchmark to know exactly when we should begin and exactly how much stretching force to use. I believe however that it is safe to do rehab strengthening exercises for at least two weeks, (at which time pain should be absent) before even the lightest of stretching is done.

But not everyone I treat is injured. Many have tight muscle structures without injury as a result of chronically bad postures or biomechanical stress. This is the point when microtrauma is affecting muscle but hasn't degraded tissue to the extent of causing true injury. These conditions are not commonly associated with substantial pain but typified by that of a low-grade ache or tension of an overloaded/overworked muscle system, (several muscles in combination trying to achieve the same goal). Imagine the muscles of the neck and upper back working in synchrony to hold up one's head that is forwardly displaced then couple this with long hours of computer or desk work.

In this instance, there is no direct injury just the accumulated stress of working day after day trying to hold an unbalanced head and stretch, massage, heat and other modalities designed to increase blood flow, oxygenation, and relaxation of muscle support structures are definitely needed. In such cases stretch should only bring comfort and no pain. If pain results from stretching either immediately or a short time following, you're dealing with a soft tissue injury! (Later you will be introduced to the Neck Correct exercise device which provides splendid therapy for tired and overworked muscles of the neck and upper back with the benefit of decreasing forward head posture.)

For healthy individuals, stretch is great to reduce muscle tension and enable an active lifestyle. However deep and overly forceful stretching should be avoided by most with the exception of highly competitive athletes who have conditioned themselves properly to allow it. Deep stretching for the average Joe or Jill can result in muscle tearing.

The Limitation of Matter

No matter how consistently we control our posture or receive the correct therapy we must still allow adequate time for rest and healing. In our fast-paced society with an emphasis on productivity, many of us simply overdo; too much, too long, too often. Injured soft tissue doesn't have to heal and over demand and overuse must be avoided. If you want to heal you have to allow for a healing environment with enough rest to ensure you can.

Common Sense is Important

Common sense is an important asset in understanding pain and injury. Some examples may help to illustrate this point:

Scenario one: You have a sudden onset of hip pain with no history of prior episodes. Your doctor sends you for x-rays of the hip and arthritic changes of the hip are seen. Your doctor reads the x-ray report from the radiologist and says your pain is due to arthritis of the hip! But wait a minute; since arthritis takes months or years to form wasn't it present two weeks ago before the onset of your pain? How could you have been pain-free all this time until now? Could you have simply strained the muscles in your hip and the arthritis be a red herring?

Scenario two: You have acute low back pain with pain in the buttock and hip with pain running down the lateral side of the leg. Your doctor requests an MRI which reveals a disc herniation or protrusion coupled with degeneration and dehydration (a gradual loss of fluid) in the disc. Your doctor says you're having low back pain and sciatica due to the disc herniation! Hold on; deteriorated discs seldom herniate! They simply don't have the mass and fullness of a healthy fluid-filled disc to be pushed out and besides, deterioration of the discs with dehydration and fluid loss takes months or years to occur. Here again, the diagnosis may be wrong. Maybe the radiologist is seeing a disc that herniated years ago and is asymptomatic. Could the fall or the snow shoveling have strained the muscles of your back and leg? Muscle tears are usually diffuse and not visible on MRI. The sciatic nerve runs down the back of the leg not the outer side of the leg. Lateral leg pain is much more likely to be a strain of the muscles and fascia on the lateral side of the leg known as TFL (tensor fasciae latae) syndrome. TFL injuries are common due to gait changes and limping will always strain leg muscles as we walk abnormally with back or hip pain! (More will be said about TFL later on.)

Scenario three: You develop chronic headaches, neck pain, possibly jaw pain as well. Your doctor says you're having migraines and loads you up on medication and possibly injections into the muscles of the neck and upper back without ever asking if you sleep on your stomach twisting your cervical spine or if you spend hours on a computer with your neck and head bent forward, creating neck and upper back strain. (A condition that leads to inflammation of the tendons and muscles of the neck inserting into the base of the skull capable of irritating the brain stem or occipital nerves often responsible for severe headache pain. This will be discussed later on.) Perhaps the TMJ pain is the result of stomach sleeping as well. With stomach sleeping the downward jaw joint is stretched while the upward joint is jammed!

Pain of any kind is seldom present without an underlying and usually fixable cause.

Always Look at Your Standing X-rays

Later in this book, we will discuss spinal x-rays and the many lapses and omissions that often accompany radiology reports. It's simply hard to believe but seldom do radiologists comment on leg length differences even large differences. Alternately when seeing a reversed or 'kyphotic' neck curvature most radiologists attribute this finding to faulty patient positioning or neck spasm which is seldom the case. (Radiologists are never in the x-ray area when technicians perform the x-ray studies so opinions concerning position and spasm are purely subjective on the part of the radiologist and have no place in reports purported to be factual!)

As crazy as it sounds you should always acquire and inspect your weight-bearing spinal x-rays. The spine assumes its true form while standing as the weight of our torsos may shift spinal components that misalign under pressure. You don't have to be a radiologist to hold your x-ray films in front of a light source or visualize digital images to determine if your hips or upper legs look level or if your neck seems to have a decent forward curve and be balanced over your erect (non-slumped) shoulder. Even a layperson can judge if a vertebra seems aligned properly with the spinal bones above and below. Don't solely depend on the verdict of the radiologist or your MD who most often only reads the radiology report. If in doubt see a competent spinal expert, a chiropractor.

Emergency Rx for Musculoskeletal Pain

Any acute presentation of muscle, joint or spinal pain could be an indication of a serious underlying problem. Although statistically unlikely, blood clots, cardiac pain, kidney stones and many other maladies can cause acute pain. So you should always consider wisely the need and indication for health provider oversight or emergency care. While true that the vast majority of acute pain is related to soft tissue injury one must use sound judgment in deciphering the need and type of care that may be indicated for your condition. When in doubt seek professional help.

If you're like most acute or chronic pain sufferers the following suggestions will be a good start to resolving your pain; first and foremost, stop stretching, massaging and vibrating the area. Switch to ice applications. (See 'Ice Is Nice' in an earlier section). See a chiropractor or chiropractic specialist to evaluate any mechanical problems that may be stressing your body. Carefully follow the postures of rest and work indicated for your condition and found in this book. Begin taking curcumin, if not contraindicated, found under 'Natural Anti-Inflammatory Aids for Healing' later in this book. Avoid any exercise in the near term until pain levels drop significantly. Reduce sugar and carbohydrate consumption (both of which may increase inflammation), and follow a good eating plan like the Mediterranean diet found later in this book. Get lots of rest and be assured that your body has an amazing and innate ability to heal itself.

Patient Scenarios

The following patient stories will help you see your painful condition in a different light, letting you identify the many incorrect practices you and 95% of all musculoskeletal pain sufferers make; damaging practices, postures and habits guaranteed to keep you in pain. Many of these patient stories occurred exactly as told, others are composites. With each, you'll learn the dos and don'ts of posture and practices, relevant to each condition; knowledge that will help to put you in the pink.

We will begin with Bob's story. While much longer than others, it accurately represents nearly half of all the patients I see, those with severe low back pain that is being improperly treated.

Bob's Low Back and 'Sciatic' Leg Pain

Bob is a sports nut who loves anything physical. He's more than proficient at his job but can't wait to hit the courts after work for a few games of racquetball then it's off to the weight room for an hour of serious weight lifting. Bob at 6'1" and 190 pounds is rock-hard solid muscle with little body fat. On the weekends this active thirty-year-old gravitates to the golf course and usually puts in a fifteen-mile bike ride as well. He's as fit as his college days when he led his rugby team to three regional championships.

Today will be a bit different. During a particularly intense racquetball match and while attempting a lunging maneuver to reach the ball, Bob feels a slight twinge in the right buttock area. With only minimal discomfort he dismisses the pain, finishes by winning the match and then proceeds to whip his opponent soundly in the third and final game. Lifting weights afterward, the buttock pain re-asserts itself with twigging pain on certain movements but the pain is nothing major and certainly doesn't limit his workout. Driving home Bob is aware of steady nagging pain in the right back and buttock. A little deep massage with his free hand seems to help a bit and some deep stretches and a hot bath at home loosen him up nicely and he falls asleep with a faint smile as he remembers his prowess in his earlier racquetball match.

Early the following morning while turning in bed, Bob is awakened by the most intense pain of his life! The pain in the back-buttock-hip and rear right thigh is searing! He lies there for a while attempting to massage and stretch the area which again seems to 'loosen' him somewhat and he can get out of bed. Again a hot shower seems to help and Bob can dress with some difficulty and sit down to breakfast. After sitting with his fiancée at the breakfast table he's unable to get out of his chair. Each attempt is meant with crushing back pain so intense that he cries out, buckling back into his seat. With increasing pain and severe 'spasms', his fiancée helps him hobble to a nearby emergency care center. There he is diagnosed with sciatica, given a shot in the buttock for muscle spasms, a prescription of hydrocodone for pain and told to go home and rest and apply a heating pad. Two days later still in bed and barely able to rise, walk of support his weight on the right leg, he is seen by his M.D. who changes the meds that are making him nauseous and tells Bob to continue the heating pad, to perform mild stretches and orders an MRI of the low back. Two days later the MRI is performed and two days following that, Bob's M.D. calls, to say that the study is negative. Bob, unable to walk more than a few steps and in severe pain is referred to a physical therapist that he sees one week later. His doctor's prescription for the PT includes moist hot packs, massage, electrical muscle stimulation and passive and active range of motion of the hip, back and leg for three weeks at three times per week. The therapist is dedicated and the sessions lengthy, lasting about an hour. The massage and stretching are painful but seem to ease the pain for a short time following each visit. Unfortunately, within an hour or two of each session, Bob tightens up again and the pain returns with a vengeance. He's given home stretches by the therapist with the same result. At the end of the three weeks of physical therapy, Bob is re-evaluated by his MD. He still has not returned to work and his general motion and comfort level have not improved. In fact, Bob is feeling worse. Now it seems that he had developed pain in his lateral thigh and calf. Two days ago he developed a wicked headache, a rare phenomenon for Bob and he is sleeping poorly. To add to the problem Bob's boss is calling, at first solicitous, but lately more demanding; "How much longer will you be out?" With bills piling up and barely able to walk with a pronounced limp due to pain, Bob loads up on pain meds and goes back to work. Sitting, driving, bending, walking and even concentrating is difficult but Bob can get through the day if he keeps up a steady flow of meds and ibuprofen.

Time passes and Bob isn't getting better, can't exercise and can't get a definitive answer about what is going on. "Well we know it's not your disc", says his M.D., "maybe you have injured the sciatic nerve?" Bob like most of us is most comfortable operating within a certain comfort zone. He has his favorite foods, people, restaurants and hangouts. He always sees his M.D. if he has a health problem. However, now he has a problem his medical doctor can't fix; what to do? In this instance, Bob talks to a co-worker and former patient in our clinic who refers him. Bob has never been to a chiropractor but has gotten to the point that he'll try anything to get relief!

Insurance coverage for each patient varies but in Bob's case, he must have a referral from his primary medical doctor, referring him to see me. With some reluctance, Bob calls his M.D. and explains the recommendation from his buddy at work and asks for the referral. Bob's M.D., wanting to give his patient every opportunity to improve, gives Bob the referral.

Day 1

Bob enters my office and completes standard intake forms regarding his specific problem given him by my receptionist. This includes his health history, work requirements, prior accidents including any surgeries, lifestyle habits, medications, family health problems, hobbies, exercise, and in short. Information that can help me understand what has happened to this young fellow and why he's not getting better. After completing the initial paperwork I call him from the waiting area and conduct him to an examining room.

However, the examination has already started! (I usually go out to the waiting room to greet new patients. This allows me to watch them rise from a chair and walk to the examining room.) Bob gets up slowly and in obvious pain as he levers himself from the chair by pushing himself erect with the strength of his arms. He is bent at the waist initially and slowly rights himself with a grimace as he begins to limp toward me. Following behind I see he has no sideward tilt of the torso that would usually be present with a herniated lumbar disc, (an involuntary tilt of the torso due to spasm of low back muscles to reduce disc pressure). He steps onto the right foot in a quick somewhat jarring fashion as he hastily attempts to transfer his weight to his left non-painful leg. Asked to sit in the examining room I note the halting manner of his slow descent into the chair and his careful attempt to guard the right side of his back and buttock. I note his placing of the right painful leg atop his left in a crossed leg attitude; a position that gives many back pain patients momentary relief!

I take a few minutes to review the intake information asking for clarifications here and there to get a basic understanding of the status of the young man before me. (Bob is squirming in the chair in serious discomfort!) I begin by checking off a long list of possible health problems and complications that could play into Bob's back pain... no history of a severe accident to the back or any surgeries? No? Okay. What was this medication you're on? I can't read his scribble. No health problems; no diabetes or history of cancer? Everything seems ordinary so far with no suggestion of an underlying disorder that could produce Bob's pain.

"Bob, did they do any lab work on you?" Lab work is a routine procedure in prolonged back pain. Both a complete CBC with morphology, (a look at the shape and nature of the blood cell composition), and a urinalysis should be performed as a basic study. More involved testing and certain blood chemistries to eliminate forms of arthritis, Lyme's disease and other conditions may be needed as well. Such testing is done to rule out less common causes of pain. Your MD or chiropractor should order these if indicated.

"They did some tests, blood and urine studies."

"Everything checks out okay?"

"Healthy as a horse," Bob says this then clenches his teeth as he shifts his position. Preliminaries over, the real work begins; Dr. Hargis plays detective.

"Okay fellow, tell me what's going on."

"Well Doc", Bob says with a sardonic smile, "my back and butt are killing me, I can't sit, I can't stand, I can't sleep, I'm barely able to walk or work, my Boss is ready to fire me, my fiancée is tired of my bitching and basically I feel like crap."

"Well Bob, I'm happy to see you haven't lost your sense of humor!"

Bob's reflexive smile and short chuckle quickly pass as the laugh brings him a brief stab of low back pain! Recovering, Bob looks up and in his eyes, I can see the fear that is the companion of every man or woman in severe pain. The message is clear; 'What the hell is going on and will I have to live like this?'

No Bob, you won't. "Okay, so how did this get started?" Bob

pauses a moment as looking down he tries to remember backward through the weeks of suffering, exams and therapy to the origins of his pain. "Well Doc, I was playing racquetball and I felt a little twinge or pull in my butt. I mean it was no big deal! But when I woke up the next morning, I guess I should say when the pain woke me up, I couldn't get out of bed. After a while I was able to make it to a nearby, 'First Care' office," and the whole story unfolds.

"Do you have a copy of the MRI?"

"No Doc."

"Did they take plain x-rays as well?"

"You bet! All fine."

"Call the facility and tell them that I'm requesting copies be sent to me. I'll give them a look just to be sure, okay? Bob, do you have any pain going down your right leg or into your foot?"

"Some in my outer leg and calf but nothing compared to my back and butt. I mean sometimes it seems to go into my leg a bit but just to the calf."

"There's no numbness in your leg?"

"No."

"You have any trouble moving your bowels, urinating or getting an erection?" A disc herniation that compresses nerves innervating the bladder, penis or bowels can alter their function. Recent fever or painful urination could indicate a bladder or kidney infection that could produce back pain but since the lab work was performed and found to be negative the chances of this are unlikely.

"No. I mean my back hurts if I strain to move my bowels but I can do it." It's normal for damaged muscles to hurt with straining.

"Good. How do you sleep? I mean what position do you favor?"

"Well Doctor Hargis, to tell you the truth, the only way I feel comfortable is lying on my stomach, my left side with a pillow between my knees or maybe my back. If I lie on my right side it kills me!" Sleeping on the bad or injured side with a muscle tear continues to stretch the muscle in that position thus worsening the injury. Often patients will state that going to bed with mild pain they were awakened from sleep in severe discomfort to find they were lying on the injured side. Because low back strain usually involves tearing of muscle tissue in the lumbar spine, hip, buttock or lower rib cage, side sleeping with the injured side of the spine curved downward, elongates damaged tissue aggravating the injury. Back sleeping with a pillow beneath the knees keeps damaged tissue shortened and linear allowing it to heal. Sleeping with the non-painful side down with a pillow between the knees is also beneficial.

"What do you do for relief or to cope with the pain?"

"Well, my therapist showed me a bunch of stretches that seem to help me a little."

"Yeah? Like what?"

"Well, I lie on my back and pull my knees to my chest or keep my upper back on the floor while I rotate my legs and knees to the side. Sometimes I lie on my stomach and bend my back as far backwards as I can."

"And what does this do?"

"Well, it loosens up my back for a while."

"What's a while?"

"Twenty minutes. Then my back tightens up again".

"Are you stretching a lot?"

"Well, every-time I feel tight, I guess I do."

"Do you take any medication?"

"My doctor gave me some pain killers but they don't do much for the pain, just make me dopey. I take ibuprofen and that seems to help for a while." (Ibuprofen is an effective pain medication because it blocks the action of enzymes released with tissue damage that would normally raise body temperature, increase swelling and make one more sensitive to the pain. Like most pharmaceutical anti-inflammatories ibuprofen can irritate the stomach and intestines causing ulcerative erosions of the stomach and intestinal walls, kidney and liver damage and other complications.)

"Do you use any heat or ice? Or perform any massage?"

"Heat feels good. I use it sometimes when it really hurts and my girlfriend gives me massages that loosen up my back and leg a little."

"Does that good feeling last?"

"Well for a while but then I seem to tighten up and the pain comes back within a half-hour or so. So I do the stretching routine again. Doc, do you mind if I stand up?" Bob pushes himself out of his chair and takes a few limping steps around the room. "My hip is killing me. I've got to move. Well, can you help me?"

"Yes. But I've got to tell you you've been wasting a lot of time up to now. Essentially, this is day one and you're starting over." From Bob's history, a negative MRI and my observations it is fairly apparent that he has experienced a soft tissue injury and has been doing everything wrong. Physical exertions like lunging for a ball while experiencing a minor jab of pain which seems to quickly pass only to intensify later on, is a story I've heard many times. My examination will likely confirm my suspicion.

"Doctor Hargis, I've been in pain for three months! I've suffered the pains of hell and now you're saying I'm just at day one?"

"Well actually Bob, I think the pains of hell are just a little more intense and this isn't the first day of your problem relived but the first day of your recovery."

I get a deep and steady gaze from Bob as he wonders if I'm crazy of if, just possibly, he's come to the right place. "Okay, so what have I got to do?

"Take your outer clothes off right down to your briefs and let me take a good look at you." Female patients receive a full-length gown that opens down the back for examination purposes while keeping their undergarments on.

Bob's petty amazing; even with three months off from his workouts he is rippling with muscle. Despite his fine physique however, he moves haltingly and with much pain. Any attempt to bend his torso or twist at the waist as he removes his clothing produces transitory jabs of intense pain that weaken his knees and nearly cause his collapse. This is a 'reflexive contraction' of damaged muscle and unlike a muscle spasm passes quickly. As Bob turns to face me I can see he is acutely embarrassed by frailty he has never known.

"Okay, turn around with your back to me and put your big toes on the green tape, hip-width apart."

I have a short piece of green tape placed parallel to the rear wall of my exam room. Bob assumes the position with his feet pretty much under his hips at about 12 inches of width apart. Even though Bob's in pain he can stand erect with no distortion or tilt of his torso. With acute disc herniations, the patient usually has a left, right or forward posture or tilt of the torso. This is especially so if the herniated disc is large enough to compress the spinal cord or spinal nerves. The fact that Bob can stand erect is further evidence, along with the negative MRI, that a disc herniation is not involved. Since Bob's condition is now three months old I ask him if he was bent initially and he denies it. Disc herniations often reduce in size with time.

As Bob maintains his standing position, I stand behind him and observe his posture. He stands erect and his pelvis appears level as well. This is important since a high proportion of low back pain sufferers have an uneven lower back, often seen when one side of the lower back appears higher than the other. This is often the case when one leg is shorter or the lumbar spine or pelvis is misaligned or abnormal in its formation. It’s good to see that Bob's low back seems to be level and balanced. I step up behind Bob and placing a hand atop both of Bob's upper hips I rotate his hips and torso gently to and fro. His back moves easily during this maneuver I call 'The Hargis Sway Test', as I rock his torso gently side to side, rotating first right then left. If Bob were having sustained spasms of the back, lasting minutes to hours, his muscles would be locked in a strong and sustained contraction making this gentle rocking impossible. This maneuver proves that Bob is not in spasm.

"Okay fellow, bend down like you're going to touch the floor." Bob begins but can only touch his knees as with bending he stretches the damaged muscles in his low back and right buttock. He grimaces on arising and tells me that to do so is more painful than the bending. (As Bob arises from his bent position his damaged back and hip muscles must work to right him. Badly strained or torn muscle tissue will produce pain on deep stretch or contraction.) Bob is also able to rotate and bend his back from side to side, but not fully and with some pain localized to the right-sided muscles.

"Show me exactly where it hurts."

Bob places his right index finger at the middle and upper area of his right buttock. "What about your spine itself?"

"Well, I get a little pain there but not as much. The majority is here and along the side of my spine." Bob points again to the thick ridge of well-developed muscles about two inches to the right of the center of his spine.

"Okay, I'm going to stress your back just a little." Stepping up to Bob once again I place my left thump firmly into the center of his lumbar spine area and grasping his right shoulder with my free hand I rock him gently backward asking him to tell me if this maneuver produces pain. Bob denies any pain in his extended and rotated spine but points clearly to the right buttock and lower back as he gasps with some added discomfort at the maneuver. This maneuver called a Kemp's test should elicit pain in the spine as well as the buttock if the spine were strongly involved. The fact that little spine pain is experienced is a good indicator that there are no significant problems with the discs or spinal vertebrae.

"Bob stand up on your toes... good. Now heels... good. And now stand on one leg close your eyes and touch your right index finger to your nose. Bob does all this and hits the mark, indicating that his central nervous system is working well and that he has no significant weakness in his legs. Leg weakness and or numbness from the back to the foot is a finding often encountered when dealing with and an injured disc that's compressing spinal nerves.

"Okay Bob, why don't you sit on the examining table and let's check your reflexes." Both the knee and ankle reflexes are brisk and normal another indicator of a healthy spine without nerve or spinal cord irritation.

"Now Bob, just raise your legs straight out in front of you." Bob does so but gets a strong twinge of pain in the right buttock which doesn't travel down his leg; a finding supporting muscle damage without nerve pressure. A herniated disc or a mechanical slippage of a lumbar vertebra compressing a nerve would tend to produce leg pain or numbness with possible loss of power in the leg.

"Bob I'd like you to take a deep breath, hold it in and strain down hard for ten seconds like you're straining to move your bowels." Bob does this and while at it I ask him to cough hard at the end. Bob completes this maneuver called 'Dejerine's Test' and I ask him if he felt any pain or numbness in the spine, back, buttock or leg. He denies pain other than in the buttock and right back muscles. Mechanical pressure on a nerve or spinal cord from a 'slipped' or herniated disc, or in some cases a misaligned vertebra, will be intensified by this test. The absence of any significant pain in the spine or running into the leg is further assurance that Bob's injury is muscular.

I grasp both of Bob's big toes in my hands and ask him to push upward with his toes against my resistance. His ability to do so in a strong fashion is further evidence of a healthy non-damaged nerve status.

Lastly, as Bob is sitting and while standing behind him, I rotate his torso. With my right fingertips placed atop Bob's lowest four spinal vertebrae, I note that two of the vertebrae seem limited in movement. This is an indication of spinal fixation of the lumbar spine. (Spinal vertebrae can become fixed in abnormal movement patterns and this is termed subluxation by chiropractors. If a subluxation is located spinal manipulation, (chiropractic adjustments), are indicated.

Asking Bob to stand I raise the examining table to an upright vertical position and ask Bob to face the table and step up slightly to a small platform at the base of the examining table as I then gently lower Bob downward to examine his back. Patients in significant pain find it difficult to move with ease and a self-righting pneumatic examining table can be a real blessing.

Once in position and with Bob resting comfortably face downward, I continue to evaluate Bob's pelvic movement and muscle tissue. Many cases of low back or buttock pain involve restriction of pelvic movement. The pelvis is a combination of three bones; the centrally located sacrum and two larger pelvic bones on either side, the innominate bones. It is the expansion of these bones at their common joints, the sacroiliac joints, that allows for the passage of a baby at birth when the innominates flex outward from the sacrum to enlarge the opening of the birth canal. Because they are flexible and assist in locomotion they can at times become subluxated acquiring fixed or aberrant motion. Fortunately, Bob's sacral joints are moving freely as I gently press downward with my palm upon each in turn and note the smooth movement of the joints and how either leg in turn slowly elongates with the motion; a normal finding.

With Bob comfortably face down I now grasp each of his heels with my hands and push firmly on each toward his head. I'm checking for equal leg length. When legs are dissimilar in length by as much as a quarter-inch or more, knee pain, hip degeneration, shin splints, scoliotic curvature in children and chronic back pain may result and injury to these areas is much more common. This is just another check for good low back balance and fortunately for Bob, his legs are even.

As I begin to more closely inspect Bob's back and buttock muscles I already have a good idea that Bob's injury is a combination of a focal restriction or 'subluxation' between two lumbar vertebrae and a muscle strain or tear. The history of a seemingly mild or even unknown trauma coupled with slowing increasing pain over several hours, followed by weeks or months of stretching or massage with no improvement or worsening of pain, is a common theme I've heard countless times from patients.

Now I place both my thumps side by side and standing above Bob and to his right I gently but deeply push into the muscle structure of the right spinal muscles. In turn, I press slowly into several areas of muscle tissue throughout the back, posterior ribs, buttock and leg muscles. Most of these deep palpations are accompanied by fairly benign reactions of only mild pain. In the muscles of the upper buttock and right lower back Bob reacts with a strong grimace of pain, withdrawing from my probing fingers as I palpate the area of torn muscle tissue which is boggy and feels swollen. Following this, I perform the same deep palpation into the area of the central lumbar spine itself. In this instance, Bob reacts with milder pain. If Bob had a significant spinal or disc problem this maneuver would elicit severe pain. Even though discs are situated forward in the spine, deep pressure into the vertebrae of the back, will also exert force and stretch into the spinal discs. A swollen or injured disc will usually be exquisitely painful with this maneuver.

Now I'm finally satisfied with my examination, the picture is complete; Bob has torn muscles in his back and buttocks coupled with spinal subluxation. Bob, like all of us, has large muscles attaching the bony structures of the spine, pelvis and leg. Due to the leverage involved in lifting objects far from the body, the muscles of this region must be large and usually quite strong. Despite their strength however, muscle, like any tissue is quite susceptible to momentary over-load or unreasonable and violent stretching. When Bob lunged for the racquetball he tore muscle and shifted the spine. This is an injury that when severe enough and with sufficient swelling in the damaged area, can irritate regional pain nerves producing exquisite discomfort. He hasn't healed because he hasn't received the right therapy for his condition which here-to-fore wasn't even understood.

It is interesting to note that the MRI did not discover the tear. Few muscle tears entail complete rupture. Most are more diffuse in nature, with a small percentage of the fibers being torn in a spread-out fashion throughout the muscle. MRI is seldom capable of imaging this very common form of trauma.

As I explain my findings to Bob, how he has injured himself and why he hasn't healed, I begin to see his eyes light in understanding. As he begins to make the connections between all those times he was stretched or was manipulated by his therapist and the pain that followed shortly after. Or the long commute to work in his slumped position when he could barely exit from the car; the times when a deep massage or hot bath seemed a blessed relief only to result in a dramatic return of his pain shortly thereafter.

"But I thought I was doing the right thing. I was doing what the therapist told me!'

"Bob I completely understand and you're not alone. The vast majority of my patients get the same bad advice. You have diffuse tearing inside contingent muscle groups coupled with spinal misalignment. The tear is a deep wound that is trying to heal. Unlike a cut on your skin, muscle fiber tears take weeks and months to heal. Every time you stretched, twisted or bent your back deeply, or sat slumped on your way to work or while watching television on your soft and sloppy couch you irritated the injured muscle more! Every time you got a massage, those torn and damaged muscle fibers were re-injured. You were essentially tearing the scab off the wound! You keep that up and I'll guarantee you'll never heal! I see patients daily that have had pain for months or years. It could be pain in the back, neck, shoulder, hip, leg, elbow you name it. The vast majority of them, have similar tissue damage and just like you have been doing the same wrong things!"

"But the heat, stretching and massage feel good!"

"They do temporarily. Massage, stretch and heat loosen damaged muscle. Stretch also sends nerve signals to the brain diminishing the brain's awareness of the pain for a time. All these maneuvers feel good but keep rewinding the clock on your healing."

"Well, I guess I've been a real horse's ass!'

"No Bob. You thought you were doing the right thing because those actions made the pain better for a while. You were doing what you thought was best."

"Well, can you help me?"

"I already have. Now you know what's wrong. You have to know that before we can make it right. Over the next few weeks, I'll help you get better. It may take several months for complete tissue healing but you should feel significantly better after just a few days as we begin to reduce swelling in the area. You'll have to do exactly as I say. Perform the therapy that I tell you to, get in here for ultrasound therapy, watch your posture and suspend any stretching, massage, heat or exercise until I tell you differently."

"You don't need to x-ray me?"

"Bob, I don't believe there's anything serious going on with your spine itself. Let's give this a week or two performing the indicated therapies and home care. By then I think you'll be a lot better. If I don't see things improving as I'd like, I'll do x-rays. Okay?"

"What about my sciatica?"

"Bob you've been limping now for weeks. Every time you came down quickly on the right leg in an attempt to get off the painful buttock/leg you shocked the muscles of the leg and hip and strained them more. You don't have sciatica and never did. You've simply been straining the leg! Hereafter, you must walk more slowly and smoothly transition your weight from side to side."

At this point I have Bob lie face down on the table. Lowering his briefs slightly I expose the injured muscular area and begin applying ultrasound. Ultrasound (US) is a wonderful therapy for healing tissue; an actual sound wave of considerable penetrating power. Not the same as its diagnostic cousin used to visualize a developing fetus or kidney stone. Ultrasound produces an extremely safe waveform that penetrates the damaged tissue with sound waves creating an acoustic effect similar to the effect of a pebble thrown into water. The sound waves generated from oscillating crystals in the ultrasound head, promote rapid passage of swelling and inflammatory products from the damaged tissue and a rapid influx of healing proteins and cellular components. Ultrasound is my therapy of choice for acute tissue injuries and its use can greatly speed up healing while diminishing the likelihood of scar formation in the damaged tissue. US is also used to soften or reduce scar tissue if already present. Just as a cut can heal with a scar so can muscular tears if the damage is severe or the injury prolonged.

While Bob relaxes enjoying this soothing and healing therapy my specially designed therapy table allows for his head and neck to be comfortably downward. This is a position also beneficial to individuals suffering from painful neck and shoulder conditions. Now seems the perfect time to tell Bob about...

Posture

"Bob, since you've torn back muscles, it's essential that you keep them short while they're healing. Standing and sitting straight is important and the posture in which your muscles are at their shortest and most relaxed. Any posture that stretches the back and elongates the muscle is going to continue to disrupt the healing tissue. Whenever you sit you've got to sit straight with your knees at or below your hips. At all costs, you've got to avoid slumping and sitting 'like a cheese curl'. This also means no floor sitting, sitting on small or low chairs, low stadium bleachers, non-supportive office or lounge chairs or with knees crossed."

"Also, all maneuvers of excessive or deep bending and twisting at the waist must be avoided. If you have to stoop, you bend your knees and squat keeping your back straight. This includes even sitting on the toilet where your back must also be straight."

"You'll have to adjust your car seat as well. Many seats have a lumbar curve but even so, the seat beneath you usually slopes downward toward the seatback. This makes it difficult to sit anyway but in a slump. If this is the case you may want to fold a dense wool blanket or large towel with extra layers toward the seatback to raise the seat to a flatter more 'bench-like' arrangement. Adjusting the seatback backward is also a good idea as this allows for some extension of the lower back. With these modifications, you may need to move the seat a little closer to the steering wheel as sitting too far away may end-up rounding out your low back as well."

"The same rules apply at work. You must sit high and straight!"

Starting to realize this process may not be a snap Bob asks. "For how long do I have to do all that".

"For as long as you sit and until you heal; weeks certainly, perhaps months. The same considerations apply to sleep. Sleep on your back with a pillow under your knees or if you have no neck or shoulder problems you can spend part of the night on your stomach if you're comfortable. If you choose this position don't raise one leg as this also produces low back stretch. Some time spent on the left side is also okay but if you're in this position you'll have to have a pillow between your legs. If the right upper leg is allowed to fall downwards so that the right inner knee touches the mattress the right hip and lateral leg can continue to be strained and overstretched even in sleep. Such a posture will also play hell with knee conditions over-stretching the entire mechanism of the knee in sleep and retarding healing." One cardinal message is made clear to Bob. Never sleep on the bad side. This position is guaranteed to continue over-stretching the torn muscles of the back and buttock. If ignored, even for a few seconds per night healing will be slow, incomplete or non-existent. Healing muscle fibers are akin to threads. How long does it take to break a thread?

As I finish the ultrasound, I place a towel over the lower back and mist it with a spray bottle of water. Now it's time to discuss a 'cool therapy'.

Ice Pack 'Cryotherapy'

"What's that?"

"A moist towel; you're getting an ice pack!"

"Ice, I don't like ice."

"Ice is nice: especially helpful for acute muscle tears. Have you tried it?

"Once but it seemed to stiffen me up more and besides my problem is three months old".

"Bob, this may have happened three months ago but for all the healing you've done, it might as well have happened yesterday. Ice is what you're getting and just one of the therapies that are going to make you better."

"How long do I ice."

"For fifteen minutes every hour or two. The ice pack is placed within a slightly moistened towel and placed directly atop the area of muscle injury. Take the ice pack right out of the freezer. It's best to use a large gel-type ice pack that's flexible and can be molded right around the damaged areas."

I carry most of the aids I recommend for my patients and will supply Bob with an ice pack before he leaves the office.

"Well I can't ice at work"

"Do the best you can when you have the time."

Although some authorities recommend ice therapy for just 48 hours following acute injury, I have found ice therapy to be effective over a much longer period. Swelling in an injured area continues for days or weeks even as the region is healing. Ice packs are an effective way to decrease swelling in acute or chronic injuries that haven't begun to mend. I advise Bob that we may want to employ the ice packs over an extended period. As I follow his progress I'll let him know when ice is no longer needed.

"What about sports, the gym?"

"No gym until I give you the go-ahead. As you heal we'll probably vary therapy slightly but absolutely no stretching or exercise until I say so. At some point, I'll also start you on a re-strengthening program that will assist the muscles in healing." Although torn tissue cannot tolerate stretch in the initial phases of healing when it is most fragile, strengthening exercises that entail muscle contraction can begin when sufficient healing has occurred. This usually corresponds to a pain level of one or two on an Analog Pain Scale,

"I'd also like you to use a lumbar spine pillow to support the back in sitting and as an aid to ensuring your continued adherence to the rules of good sitting posture." A lumbar pillow will provide support for Bob's injury which he will have prior to leaving the office. Finishing Bob's 15 minutes of ice pack application and with the back somewhat 'numb' according to Bob, I tell him I would like to perform a gentle spine adjustment or manipulation, explain the procedure and with his consent we proceed.

Spinal Manipulation

Positioning Bob on his side with the upper leg slightly bent I gently stretch the lower back as a low but just audible series of three small pops is heard. This manipulation will improve spinal mobility and assist in re-establishing proper spinal mechanics. The maneuver elicits some mild pain in the muscle tissue but is slight compared to what Bob experiences with each shift of his body. The force of the manipulation is mild as excessive force or stretch could be damaging to the healing tissue.

Some people fear the very thought of having their back ‘cracked', a derogatory term for the sound produced when spinal joints similar to the type of joints found in the fingers are stretched. Feeling the ease and lack of pain associated with spinal manipulation when performed by a licensed DC, is the best way to dispel their anxiety. In my opinion, no other health provider should manipulate the spine as they significantly lack a chiropractor's expertise. This may be the only time I adjust Bob in the near term or we may do adjustments periodically as his pain and swelling remiss. Generally, in the early stages of a muscular injury, that does not heavily involve issues within the spine itself, it is best to avoid excessive or frequent spinal manipulation.

Of all major health care providers, chiropractors pay the smallest malpractice premiums in the country. This relates directly to the safety of their treatment. Gentle spinal manipulation, even in many cases of disc herniation, is safe and can be highly effective in restoring proper spinal function.

As I raise the table Bob rides upward to an erect position, steps gingerly from the table and moves slowly in a testing fashion. He continues with obvious pain but states he may feel just a bit better.

The Tie That Binds

"Is that it?"

"One last thing," I bend down removing a small white box from the bottom of the exam room cabinet and I withdraw an elastic and Velcro low back support belt. "Bob those with muscular tears of the lower back need back support. Wearing a lumbar support snugly in the initial stages of healing will make an immense difference in the way you feel. Short-term use won't weaken your back and if worn properly, will support injured muscles, diminish back pain and assist healing. I'd like you to try it."

Bob complies as I help him to position and tighten the support belt properly. Once in place, the effect is immediate. Bob smiles broadly as he moves guardedly about the room.

"Damn, this feels pretty good. I could have used one of these weeks ago."

"You could have used a lot of things a few weeks ago but we'll just have to be satisfied with doing the right things now."

Finishing, I give Bob a sheet of instructions to recap the dos and don'ts discussed and advise him to rest, ice and follow all the instructions carefully. I ask him to set-up appointments three times per week for the next four weeks and tell him I have every confidence in his impending improvement provided he follows the game plan.

"One last word of caution; we did a lot today Bob, a lot of poking, prodding and examination. Don't be surprised if you're just a bit sorer tomorrow. Also, it will take two to four days for the swelling to start to decrease now that you're following the correct path. Since your tissue swelling is directly proportional to the degree of your pain it will also take two to four days to begin seeing a reduction in your pain and that will happen only if you are doing exactly as told. Be patient over the next few days and call me if you should need anything prior to your next visit."

Bob looks me straight in the eye saying, "Thanks, Doctor Hargis. I really appreciate the time and the way you explained everything. I feel a lot better now just knowing where I stand."

Bob now understands his injury and has been given a solid plan for healing and a general timeline for improvement. He is now a happier, less confused and less fearful individual; a mental state much more conducive to healing than the one with which he entered my office.

Week Four and Bob is Ready for Rehab

Bob is recovering nicely with regular spinal adjustments and proper therapy. He presents with good back motion and a level of 1 or 2 pain on the analog scale. It's time to begin rehab exercise and I instruct him in core exercises for the back, stomach and hamstrings.

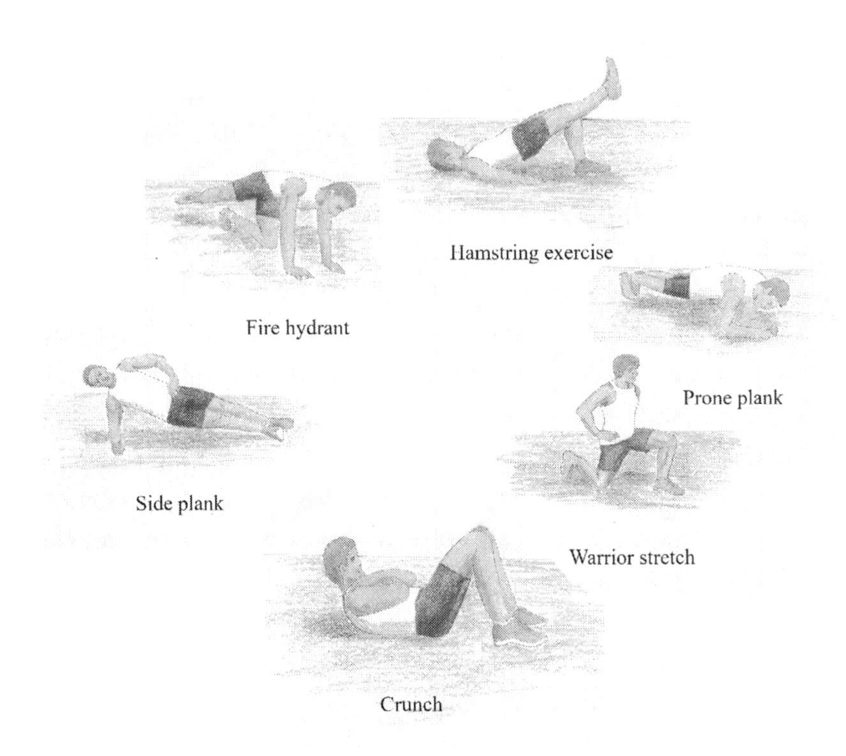

Exercise here cannot be rushed or overdone. A few light reps done on day-one are followed by adding just one or two more repetitions of each exercise the following day if you are not unduly sore. If so, skip a day to recover and do the exercises on day three. At the point that exercises can be done daily without increasing pain one or two repetitions may be added each day. Each exercise should be done until the muscle groups doing the work are tired and your common sense lets you know that more could begin to strain the area. This is crucial since many people try to rush rehab and relapse. It's always better to be under the guidance of a trained health care professional when performing rehab and these are only general guidelines. As strength develops increase reps to a point that several repetitions of each exercise can be accomplished easily. This may take up two to four weeks. Generally, it is at this point, when the exercises become easy and the injured area is completely non-painful that one can consider a very gentle and gradual stretching program. I usually advise that the patient be pain-free and continuing ultrasound therapy for at least two weeks before doing even the lightest stretching. When doing so, caution is needed, while slowly increasing range of motion over days or weeks. Care must be given to a slow sports re-integration as well, at reduced efforts initially while building to full capacity over time. Listen to your body! It will tell you when you can begin to increase time and intensity.

Rehab exercise should never begin when analog pain scale numbers are high. I usually recommend waiting until the pain has reduced to an analog scale of 1 or 2. Some authorities like to start a bit sooner but you run the risk of exacerbating the injury if healing tissues lack sufficient strength to withstand the rehab exercises. The biggest mistake is going too hard, too fast and too soon. Listen to your body and remember that rehab is initially about contracting muscle only; stretch comes later when healing is far advanced.

Visit HealingTheHumanMachine.com for a video demonstrating my preferred low back rehab exercises.

Sandra's Neck Pain and Headaches

Sandra, a night duty nurse and mother of four, is constantly on the go. Unable to ever relax she arrives home from her shift at a local hospital in time to say goodbye to her husband Carl departing for his 'day job', prepares breakfast and lunches for her two younger children who are finicky eaters and mediates the ongoing disputes between her two twin teens. Beset by money issues this forty-something Mom is plagued by constant tension in the upper back and shoulders. She knows she holds herself too tightly but seems unable to relax as she is plagued by concerns of finances and family. After she puts the kids to bed, she likes to read a little and will usually prop herself up in bed with several pillows to do so. Lately, her tension headaches have been worsening and she has constant neck pain and soreness especially at the base of her skull. In the last two weeks, she has begun to have pounding pain from her upper neck and rear skull coming over the head and into her right temple. (With a normal blood pressure that she checks herself she knows that the headaches are not due to high blood pressure.)

Sandra is sleeping poorly and her doctor has conjectured that she may be experiencing fibromyalgia stating that this is, 'a mysterious form of muscle pain whose nature is not fully understood' and has prescribed Paxil, a potent anti-depressant anti-anxiety drug, (with a long list of possible side effects), for her treatment. Sandra has little time for exercise, is barely able to keep up with the house and kids, feels exhausted all the time, has that dammed headache again, takes two Tylenol, smokes a cigarette and heads for bed. She'll likely continue to relive the same sequence of stress and pain day after day as her condition deteriorates and she is progressively placed on stronger (more dangerous) medications to relieve a growing constellation of diagnosed medical problems, many of which may be created by the ever-increasing complex interactions of these drugs.

Unfortunately, neither Sandra nor her doctors understand that she is experiencing the most common form of muscle injury. The common irritation and deconditioning that befalls many of us whose muscles are constantly under tension. Worsening the problem, she constantly stretches her neck, has Carl give her a massage when they have time together and occasionally wakes up on her stomach. Last week she began to sleep on two pillows as the higher position seemed to relieve the pain somewhat but now the headaches are waking her up at night.

During her last doctor's visit, he reviewed the results of the brain MRI and cervical x-rays he ordered. Everything checks out as normal except on x-ray it is noted that Sandra exhibits early degenerative changes of the spine with some disc thinning and arthritic changes of the joints. Also noted is a loss of normal forward cervical spine curve. The reading radiologist attributes this to faulty positioning during the x-ray exam or possibly spasm of the neck although he wasn't present during the x-ray and never examined Sandra. Her M.D. then suggests physical therapy and writes her a script for six weeks of therapy consisting of massage, electrical muscle stimulation, exercise and stretching. She attends a few sessions but the pain becomes worse and she discontinues therapy. A couple of her nurse friends are patients of mine and finally convince her to give me a try.

As I take the history and ask her what she does to relieve her symptoms, I can see that Sandra is a definite Type A personality. She sits, shifts and moves quickly having little patience for the delay as she taps her hand on her leg. I also take note of all the mistakes she has been making, stretch and massage, if like 95% of my patients she has soft tissue issues of the neck and upper back.

"Sandra you've been having this neck pain and more recently headaches starting about twelve weeks ago."

"That's right."

"No trauma, no falls, no heavy lifting, no extreme sports?"

"No, and my only extreme sport is folding laundry." In my experience patients with a sense of humor haven't been psychologically diminished by their pain. They do better in therapy versus individuals overly depressed and fearful about their prospects of recovery.

"Never had headaches or neck pain before?"

"No."

"OK," I explain the analog scale and she states her pain varies between a 4 to an 8 when the headaches become more extreme.

"Let's do an exam. I'm going to leave the room and I want you to put on this gown with the opening in the back. Take off your blouse, leave on your bra and pants."

When gowned I re-enter: "Could you stand up for me close your eyes and stand on one leg." She does so with good balance and control. "Okay put your foot down and lean your head back to look at the ceiling and touch your right index finger to your nose": again, accomplished neatly. "Okay, look straight ahead." Pupils are normal and symmetrical in size and narrow to focus on my finger held closely. I do a few other simple neurological tests to rule out any likelihood of brain pathology.

"Okay let me just take a moment and let me look at your posture." Posture is normal from the rear, even hips, straight spine, head erect with no right or left tilt, shoulders equal with the right side in this right-handed woman slightly lower; a normal finding. "Fine now turn and let me see your posture from the side."

Warning bells go off as I see that Sandra carries her head far forward of a normal balanced position. The head should be balanced over the mid-shoulder but in Sandra's case the ear canal, the weight-bearing center of the head, is at least three inches forward of its normal balance point. This forward head carriage requires the muscles of the neck and upper back to work much harder to hold up Sandra's ten-pound head. In fact, for every inch forward of balanced head position these muscles have to double, triple and quadruple their workload; easily understood if we envision the ease of holding a bowling ball held balanced over the elbow or the increasing effort required to hold the ball leaning outward and away. As you go forward of the balance point the force required to hold the bowling ball increases dramatically. Although Sandra has only recently begun to experience neck pain the muscles of the neck and upper back have been under significant stress for years as this is a long-standing postural problem. This condition makes it much easier to strain the muscles of the neck and upper back. I explain this all to Sandra.

"Sandra I'd like you to sit here." I indicate one of my treatment tables. "I'm going to gently palpate your neck and do some orthopedic maneuvers to get a better idea of the problem." I begin to lightly touch the muscles of the neck on either side of the spine and as I do, I can feel the swelling in the tissue; even with light pressure Sandra winces and states pain. The same finding is present in the area of the upper and inner shoulder blades known as the intra-scapular region. As I palpate upward with my fingers along the spine to lightly probe the upper neck and base of the skull, pressure here produces pain that travels into the temple area where she has been experiencing her headaches. This is a strong indicator that the headaches are being generated from the neck region; a condition known as 'cervicogenic headache', the most common form of headache.[68] Some simple orthopedic maneuvers of the neck and head give me further proof of the headaches being linked to her neck pain. I explain all this to Sandra. Asking Sandra to look down, upward, move her head laterally side to side and to rotate both left then right, I see that she can rotate her head fully 85 degrees to the left but only 75 degrees to the right which causes her pain on the right side of her neck.

My palpation has also revealed that Sandra has a badly misaligned cervical spine. Instead of having a normal forward or lordotic curve of the neck she has a reversal of the curve with generalized misalignment of her spinal vertebrae. I explain this to Sandra and advise her that we will begin with therapy initially to reduce her inflammation and begin spinal adjustments to the neck as her neck tenderness and swelling decrease.

"So, you're saying my headaches are related to my neck pain?

"Absolutely, you have a negative brain MRI and you have no clinical indication of anything awry with the neurological testing I just performed. You do however have considerable inflammation of the muscles in your neck and attaching to your shoulder blades and upper ribs. These muscles are stressed having to hold your head far forward of its normal position. The referral of pain to the temple, when I palpate the base of the skull at the upper neck, is a clear marker for headaches generated from the cervical spine. The great majority of headaches including migraine and cluster headaches are cervicogenic in nature; that is to say, they arise from problems in the neck."

"So where do we go from here."

"No more stretch or massage. Every time you do that you're irritating the muscle tissues in the neck and upper torso responsible for the neck and headache pain. Use cold packs at home, 15 minutes every hour or two when possible, on the neck and base of the skull. No reading in bed with pillows propping you up and pushing your head forward. In fact, I would like you to avoid looking down as much as possible as this is only going to add more stress to your already inflamed and irritated neck muscles. When you're charting during your nursing hours, I want you to do your very best to elevate the written material and to raise your computer screen, again so you don't have to look down. You may be able to attach a paper holder to the side of your monitor. Use one pillow not two and sleep on your back. Absolutely no stomach sleeping and since your neck and intra-scapular pain is bilateral, (she has pain on both sides of her neck and shoulder blades), you have to try your best to stay off your sides as well."

"How long will it take to get better?"

"I believe that if you do as I say you'll be much better in three to four weeks. At the point when your pain scale number has dropped to a 3 or 4, we'll begin spinal adjustments and when the pain is at a 1 or 2 you'll begin an exercise program. The combination of spinal manipulation and exercise should restore your neck posture and re-balance your head properly."

Stated somewhat doubtfully, "You can do that?"

"Very likely but we're going to need to look at those x-rays your doctor ordered. We'll begin preliminary treatment consisting of ultrasound followed by ice packs today. I want you in for therapy three times a week for four weeks. No manipulation will be performed until I've had a look at the x-rays. After that, we'll begin spinal adjustments if indicated as swelling reduces. Although the radiologist indicated some early arthritic changes that would not contraindicate spinal manipulation. Adjustments of the spine will help normalize your spinal function and alignment and achieve a more normal range of motion when you attempt to turn your head to the right." Sometimes I choose to manipulate or 'adjust' a patient's spine before I see x-rays. This is simply a judgment call born out of my clinical exam and many years of experience.

"One more thing, you should really try to stop smoking. Smoking decreases blood supply and oxygen to all your tissues including your spinal discs and will slow your healing if you continue."

Last on my agenda, I tell Sandra about the benefits of a natural and powerful antioxidant/anti-inflammatory known as curcumin. We age to a large extent by oxidation and inflammation of our body tissues. Curcumin, an active neutraceutical in turmeric, reacts to reduce these damaging processes. In long term inflammation, curcumin will be beneficial to Sandra's healing without damaging her kidneys, liver, stomach or intestines as many over the counter NSAIDs do like ibuprofen, aspirin, etc. I ask her to take 95% pure curcumin each day for the next four weeks along with a little black pepper while adding fruit like blueberries or strawberries and a handful of nuts or perhaps avocado which will enhance its action. (Curcumin may react negatively when combined with certain medications and your pharmacist or physician should be consulted. We will discuss curcumin in detail later.)

Sandra's Second Visit

"Well, it's been two days. How do you feel?"

"You know I actually felt a little better after the ultrasound and ice and the ice packs at home have helped to control the headaches a little but I had a bad one this morning."

"Don't worry that's normal and this is going to take some time. As long as you can honestly say you're feeling progressively better each week we'll both be happy." I ask to examine the x-rays ordered by her M.D. It should be understood that her doctor, as in most cases, has not seen her x-rays but only the report from the radiologist. (Most M.D.s have no training to interpret x-ray studies.)

As I look at the x-ray films, I see that Sandra has a severe reversal of the neck's normal spinal curve. This abnormal curve reversal is known as a 'kyphosis'. Sandra is not alone. Many of the people I see for complaints of neck, upper back, TMJ and headache pain, have a reversed abnormal curvature of the cervical spine. Accidents, stomach sleeping, birth injuries of the neck and long hours of head flexion in study and work can affect neck posture. Although kyphosis is rarely related to spasm, when seen on x-ray, many radiologists incorrectly believe that a reversed spinal curvature is related to poor patient positioning by the technician or spasm of the patient's neck. This is a huge disservice to a large percentage of pain sufferers as a treatable condition goes undiagnosed. (Spasm of the neck is extremely rare and usually only seen in cases of extreme trauma possibly with spinal fracture. Furthermore, radiology staff are responsible for patient positioning and the medical radiologist is seldom if ever present when x-rays are taken. After having this opinion given by one radiologist on several studies I asked if he felt his staff was universally incompetent. After that he agreed to admit there might be natural causes.)

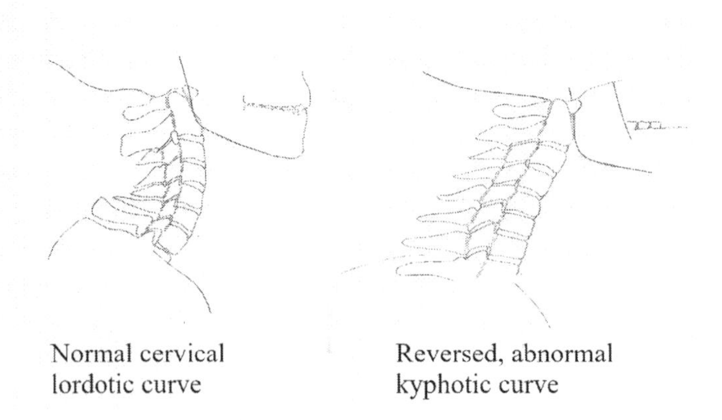

Normal cervical lordotic curve

Reversed, abnormal kyphotic curve

I show Sandra an example of a proper 'lordotic' cervical spine curve and how this allows the head to be better balanced on the torso and explain the ramifications of forward head carriage. After questioning me about restoring the curvature, I mention the device we will be using and give her a brief look at the 'Neck Correct'. I also remind her that her neck is still much too painful and inflamed to begin the mildly strenuous exercise regimen related to the device;

which will begin a few weeks from now.

Before parting, I ask about diet and exercise. "Sandra the Mediterranean diet is an excellent diet to reduce both weight and inflammation. The Mediterranean diet emphasizes eating primarily plant-based foods, such as fruits and vegetables, whole grains, legumes and nuts; replacing butter with healthy fats such as olive oil and canola oil and using herbs and spices instead of salt to flavor foods. Please look into it. Also, try to get more exercise as well, I recommend walking at least 30 minutes a day and work doesn't count. Stay away from sugar and non-complex carbohydrates as they turn into sugar quickly and increase inflammation. Check out the 'glycemic index' and learn which carbs to avoid. Try to stay away from any carb with a score above 50." More will be discussed on the subject.

Sandra's Fourteenth Visit...Week Five...On to the 'Curve Restorer/Neck Correct' Exercise Device

Sandra is now a 1 on the analog pain scale. She hasn't had a headache in two weeks and her neck pain is substantially reduced. She's been receiving spinal adjustments and doing what I asked her to do, both in in-office therapy and at home and now we will begin the cervical exercises. The 'Neck Correct or Curve Restorer' is a simple exercise device that anyone can use at home. A few minutes a day can reduce forward head carriage, restore better head balance and enhance normal lordotic curve in as little as six to twelve months. Moreover, it is a wonderful rehab took for arthritic and overworked necks in that it can strengthen the musculature of the neck and upper back, relieve neck and upper back tension and rehabilitate, to some extent, the ravages of injury and spinal degeneration involving discs and joints. (More will be said about this device later on.)

Sandra... Month Seven... Six Months with the 'Neck Correct'

I haven't seen Sandra in four months now as she was released from all care when she was four weeks pain-free. She states she feels great and has been following my advice on exercise and diet losing over twenty pounds. Today she enters with a big hopeful smile and a follow-up lateral x-ray of the cervical spine. We'll compare this to her initial x-ray taken some months ago.

Placing both x-rays side by side I see that Sandra now has a modest forward curve measured at a positive 11 degrees. Although this is less than the 30-35 degrees I believe is optimal she has improved greatly from the reversed and negative 8-degree curvature seen on the original x-ray films. A gain of 19 degrees is good progress and I tell her to keep it up and see me in another six months for a comparative study when I fully expect to see improving curvature. Later we will explore reversed spinal curvature of the neck and its effect on head position and Pandora's box of painful conditions it causes.

Visit HealingTheHumanMachine.com for a video demonstrating the Neck Correct exercise regimen or to order one.

Martin's Pinched Nerves

Martin is a middle school science teacher who after bending to retrieve lab supplies for his students forgot that an upper cabinet was open and while standing struck the back of his head soundly. With mild neck discomfort, he finished his day. Neck pain continued and within a week he began to lose feeling in both his hands which compelled him to take a leave from his position. Initial cervical spine x-rays requested by his M.D. were taken and read as normal by a medical radiologist. Following three weeks with no improvement and both a negative MRI of the cervical spine and of the brain he was referred for physical therapy but discontinued mid-way through a six-week protocol with no improvement. Returning to his M.D., he was referred to a pain specialist and a carpal tunnel surgeon. Coming from a science background, Martin suspected his neck pain had to be related to his hand numbing and had made an appointment to be seen in our office.

Entering the clinic with scans in hand, he had difficulty raising his head to look at me and stated that this flexed neck position was the only way he could find some relief from both the neck pain and hand numbing. Following my review of his cervical MRI, I found myself agreeing with the radiologist's opinion of a negative study but the cervical spine x-ray was a very different matter. This study demonstrated significant rotational subluxations of both the C5 and C6 cervical vertebrae. My palpation of his neck confirmed the continued malalignment of these vertebrae and deeper probing here provoked significant pain that radiated outward toward the extremities.

Since the spinal nerves emanating from the neck control sensation to the arms and hands it was fairly evident that we had found the source of the problem. Rotational or other forms of spinal mal-alignment can stretch and/or compress exiting spinal nerves with profound consequences. Completing my exam, I explained to Martin that in my opinion some healing therapy was indicated but more importantly, that spinal manipulation would be required to correct the rotation misalignment of the two adjacent vertebrae and relieve the hand numbness. With his permission, we began a course of cervical spine manipulation. I am happy to say that three weeks later and following ultrasound therapy and eight cervical spine adjustments Martin was once again back with his students, out of pain, with good hand function, an erect stance and remembering to always close the upper cabinet door!

Ronnie's Shoulder Pain

Ronnie's a big kid and as he sits beside his mother I marvel at his 6'6" frame at his tender age of sixteen and the size 14 shoes he wears.

I turn to his mother, "Boy, they're growing them big these days! So how can I help?"

Ronnie's mom laughs briefly and they both begin to explain the persistent right shoulder pain that has benched this aspiring young athlete in the middle of his basketball season. It seems the pain began after Ronnie's jump shot was blocked by another player. Mild at first the pain over the past four weeks has intensified greatly and now is traveling into the right arm with some tingling and numbness. The family M.D. took a look and said he thought Ron has strained the shoulder and to stretch and use ice packs. He prescribed an anti-inflammatory as well but Ronnie can't take the medication due to the stomach pain it produces. Stretching seems to help but the pain is getting worse and now in the past week the arm pain began.

"Ronnie's really special. He's a great player and we're hoping for a basketball scholarship."

I can see a lot of worry in both their eyes as Ronnie levers his right arm across his chest, grasping the right elbow with his left hand and giving the shoulder a huge stretch.

"Ron, stop that." Ronnie looks like he got his hand caught in the cookie jar.

"What?"

"No more stretching." They both look at me as if I had two heads but I'm used to that. I explain the principle of soft tissue trauma and the detriment of stretch for a condition that's probably a soft tissue injury.

"Ron, let's take a look at your posture. Take off the shirt, kick off the shoes and stand up."

Complying, I see that Ronnie is well balanced and completely normal in his posture except for some puffiness or swelling about the inner and upper aspects of the right shoulder blade or scapula.

Palpating the area at the inner margins of the scapula there is swelling noted and Ron withdraws from my lightly probing fingers as he experiences pain. Asking Ron to sit, I motion the shoulder to judge his capacity for movement and check the strength of the right shoulder and arm. All seems normal except for a little weakness when I ask Ronnie to resist my downward force on his arm while held straight out to his side. Resistance to this maneuver reduplicates his pain which he identifies as being inside and on top of his shoulder blade. (The vast majority of rotator cuff tears present with pain at the exact upper and outer corner of the shoulder. Not around the shoulder blade.) I also check his arm reflexes and do some orthopedic maneuvers to rule out any spinal complications or shoulder tendon impingement that might be present with rotator cuff issues. Everything is normal.

"Ronnie, in what position do you sleep?"

Mom chips in, "He almost always sleeps on his sides or stomach."

"And where is his arm when he's on his stomach."

His mom thinks about it, "Well, I would say probably under his pillow."

"Did his doctor ask how Ronnie slept?"

"I don't... no, he didn't."

"Okay, well the good news is that we'll probably be watching Ronnie on TV one day. I agree with Ronnie's M.D., he does have a muscle strain, however, you don't stretch a muscle strain and you don't", I turn to Ronnie, "sleep on the painful side or with the arm on that side above your head. Either will overstretch the damaged muscles attached to the inner shoulder blade as it moves away from the spine. The rotator cuff tendons will be pinched and stretched as well."

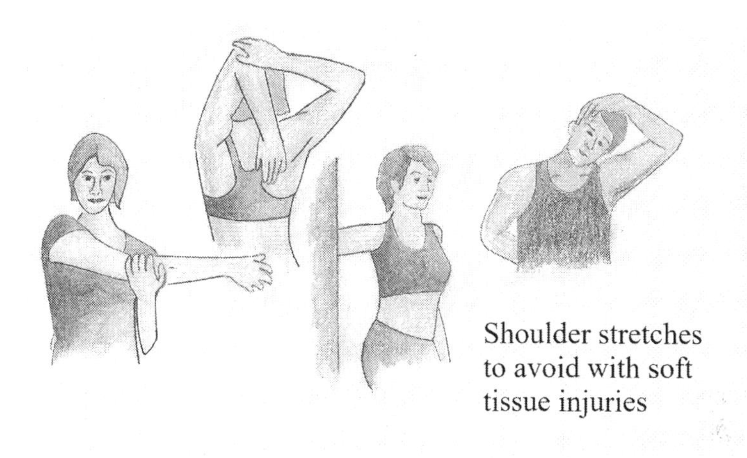

Shoulder stretches to avoid with soft tissue injuries

I explain it all to mother and son and we begin the first step of healing; educating the patient. I advise both on the dos and don'ts; ultrasound, ice and strengthening when appropriate while avoiding stretch, massage, goading or vibration of the area.

"But my coach makes me do the stretches with the rest of the team even though I can't play right now."

"I'll give you a note for the coach Ron. You'll be out for at least six weeks but if you do as I say you'll be back in the game shortly thereafter."

Ronnie Week Four... Exercise Begins

Ronnie is much better. He presents with excellent arm and shoulder motion and complaints of level 1 pain on the analog scale only occasionally and is often completely pain-free. It's time to begin rehab exercise and I instruct him in resistance band exercises, using a very light stretchable band while performing several maneuvers to strengthen the shoulder, arm and upper back.

Exercise here cannot be rushed or overdone. A few light reps done on day one are followed by adding just one or two more repetitions of each exercise the following day if you are not unduly sore. If so, skip a day to recover and do the exercises on day three. At the point that exercises can be done daily without increasing pain one or two repetitions may be added each day. As you progress, each exercise should be done until the muscle groups doing the work tire and your common sense lets you know that more could begin to strain the area. This is crucial since many people try to rush rehab and relapse. It's always better to be under the guidance of a trained health care professional when performing rehab and these are only general guidelines. As strength develops increase reps to a point that twenty to thirty of each exercise can be accomplished easily. This may take several weeks. This is generally the point that one can consider re-entering their chosen sport. When doing so care must be given to a slow re-integration at reduced efforts to build to full capacity over time. Listen to your body! It will tell you when you can begin to increase time and intensity.

Visit HealingTheHumanMachine.com for a video demonstrating my preferred shoulder rehab exercises.

Further Considerations for Shoulder Pain

While shoulder strain is by far the most common source of shoulder pain, arthritis, bursitis and rotator cuff injuries are not uncommon. Using some common sense is the best way to proceed. If a painful shoulder is usable with a fair to good range of motion and reasonable strength then waiting four to six weeks while using the strategies discussed above should help to reduce pain and improve function. Following this therapy regimen alone could be sufficient to allow healing followed by a home rehab regimen with strengthening exercises.

Arthritis

If shoulder pain is severe and there is a significant limitation of shoulder function then diagnostic tests such as x-ray and possibly MRI are in order. Arthritis and rotator cuff tears vary by degree and mild to moderate arthritis of the shoulder often responds to rest, the non-compressive and non-stretching postures I endorse along with ultrasound therapy. In cases of arthritis, a heating pad may be substituted for ice, however ice packs often work just as well. Mild cases of arthritis often respond well to moderate rehab exercise; (videos cited above). Severe cases of arthritis or bony impingement of the shoulder demonstrated on x-ray or MRI, may require surgical intervention and this should be discussed with a competent orthopedic surgeon.

Rotator Cuff Injuries

Rotator cuff injuries run the gamut from simple bruising of the rotator cuff tendons, mild strain with minimal tendon damage to complete rupture or tear of one or more tendons. The rotator cuff (RC), is composed of four muscles, the supraspinatus, infraspinatus, teres minor and subscapularis which have tendons that attach to the upper portion of the upper arm bone (the humerus). The supraspinatus arising from the upper shoulder blade thins down to become a tendon that passes between an overhanging lateral bony projection of the shoulder blade (the acromion) and the topmost portion of the ball-shaped head of the upper arm or humerus. Unfortunately, the space between the acromion and the top of the humerus is narrow and the supraspinatus tendon can be squeezed or 'pinched' when one elevates the arm laterally away from the body. This makes it the most vulnerable component of the rotator cuff. The infraspinatus and teres minor rotate the arm outward, while the subscapularis rotates the arm inward.

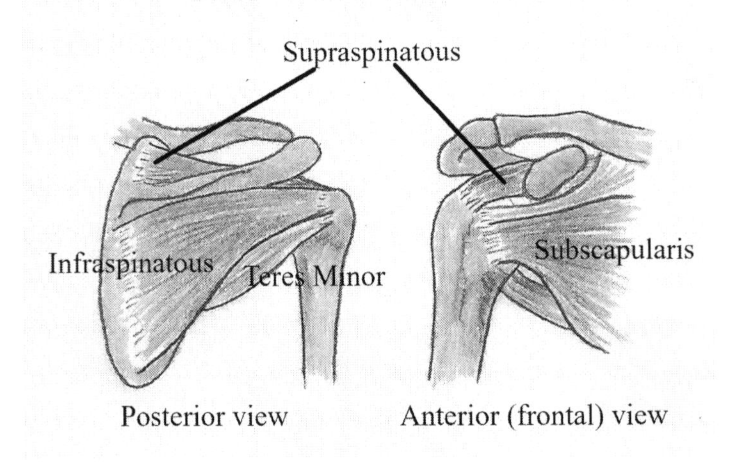

Rotator cuff tendinitis occurs when the tendons are injured, usually as a result of repetitive pinching due to overhead reaching, pushing, or lifting with outstretched arms. Athletes who perform an overhead activity, such as swimming, tennis, throwing, golf, weightlifting, volleyball, and gymnastics are also at high risk. Many injuries are the result of a fall, direct blow, or a rapid and forceful use of the arm. Tendinitis associated with a minor injury and little tearing usually responds well to the regimen discussed previously for shoulder strains.

Persistent shoulder/upper arm pain especially when coupled with limited shoulder function calls for diagnostic imaging. MRI is the best method of accessing RC injuries. Tendinitis and mild to moderate tears may be handled conservatively. In some cases, injection of a steroid may be required. More severe tears will usually require surgery. One of the first things to consider in treating a rotator cuff issue is to identify the major factors that contributed to the injury. A careful inventory of past events, work habits or postures and getting a good biomechanical assessment/physical examination is important. Based on the results, an individualized treatment plan can be designed. Interventions may include:

- Ergonomic adjustments to keep the arm less elevated; placing monitors, keyboards, and chairs at appropriate heights
- Postural retraining to improve sitting, sleeping and standing postures to reduce bowing of the shoulders can decrease 'impingement' or pinching, of the supraspinatus tendon
- Exercises for the back and inner-shoulder blade muscles, shoulder and cervical spine to improve shoulder mechanics

Liam's Headaches

Liam is a lovely little boy, ten years old and as smart as a whip: straight A's all the way! Unfortunately, Liam has a problem. Beginning about nine months ago he is experiencing migraine-like headaches almost daily, which may strike at any time and last for hours. This studious young man is now having trouble in school and his mother is beside herself with worry. She has taken Liam to two different headache specialists, spending hours in consultations and testing. With no answers or relief, the doctors want to put this child on Depakote to control his headaches! Depakote is a strong drug used to control seizures, psychiatric conditions and migraine headaches. Depakote's milder side effects include diarrhea, constipation, upset stomach, dizziness, drowsiness, weakness, hair loss, blurred or double vision, enlarged breasts, ringing in the ears, tremors, balance issues, weight gain and unusual or unpleasant taste of foods. More serious side effects include signs of infection with fevers, sore throat and swollen lymph nodes, chest pain, easy bruising, unexplained bleeding, irregular heartbeat, swelling of hands and feet, uncontrolled eye movement, shivering, rapid breathing and loss of consciousness!

Liam's mother is naturally hesitant to expose her child to these risks and has consulted with me as a last hope based on her good response to prior treatment in my office. After taking a careful history, during which I learn that brain scans and clinical examinations have been consistently normal, I ask Liam to disrobe down to his underpants and I take a careful look at this young boy. Asking him to stand on a strip of tape placed parallel to the wall of my examining room and with his back to me, feet hip-width or 8 inches apart (less than I would use for an adult), I examine his posture.

The first thing I see and somewhat surprising is that Liam tilts his head and neck toward his right shoulder. Further the ridge of muscle supporting his head on the left side of his neck is overdeveloped, tight and painful to my finger palpation. Stepping away my gaze travels downward where I see that his lower back is not level, the left pelvic crest is lower than that of the opposite right side. The difference is roughly 1/2 inch. Asking Liam to lay face down on my examining table I simultaneously press upward on the bottom of each foot where I see the level of the sole of the left foot rises approximately 1/2 inch above the right sole. Pointing this out to Liam's mom, I gently palpate and motion joints in the pelvis and lower back to check for ease of movement. Finding no fixation in spinal or pelvic movement I next examine his neck and cervical spine in more detail. The muscles along the rearward left side of the neck, just below the skull, are extremely tight and swollen. Liam lets me know, that my deep finger pressure here, produces radiating pain upward into his forehead on the left.

"Liam, does that forehead pressure feel like the headaches you get?

"Yes, it really hurts the left side of my head and around my left eye." While palpating Liam's neck I also feel a shift in the position of the uppermost cervical vertebra, the atlas, which is abnormally positioned. I ask Liam's mother to feel the neck as well and when she does Liam again expresses pain to her deeper touch.

Directing my question to his mother I ask, "Can you feel the difference side to side; the muscle tension and that the bones beneath the muscles seem more prominent on the left?"

Wide-eyed she nods her head.

I ask Liam to once again stand on the parallel tape while asking his mother to stand from behind to observe his posture as I begin to explain to both Liam and mom, that Liam carries his head tilted to the right to balance his head and torso. "In addition to a leg length difference, Liam is experiencing a left cervical muscle strain as these muscles have to work harder when he shifts his head to the right to better balance himself over his right longer leg. He also has a subluxated or shifted atlas vertebra situated just below the skull. This is common with prolonged postural stress and will require some muscle therapy and gentle spine adjustments to reposition the vertebrae. This will help to lessen the pain, improve spinal movement, better balance the spine and reduce his headaches."

Those with leg length differences must alter their posture to maintain balance. This is an unconscious and automatic balancing action of the human body. Liam does have a slight curvature of his spine toward the left short leg side but this is simply a 'balancing' or functional curve. Luckily the leg length difference doesn't appear to have caused any deformity in the shape of his spinal vertebrae which would indicate a structural scoliosis. Liam has dodged a bullet that many children do not. (More will be said about scoliosis later on.)

Differences in leg length are fairly common occurring in 13-15% of the population.[69] (Many authorities think this number is much higher.) Unfortunately, this little boy with his shorter left leg has been carrying his head to the right as a counterbalance. This has placed tremendous strain on his neck and is likely causing the headaches. Although I can't be sure, I pose this as being a possibility and suggest we formulate orthotics for Darin to equalize the height of the left leg should standing x-rays confirm the same discrepancy in leg length that my clinical exam has demonstrated.

Asking Liam to lay face-up on my adjusting table, I give him a gentle spinal adjustment to better position his shifted atlas vertebra. This is a 'tractive' type of spinal manipulation and is extremely safe. I advise his mother to place an ice pack on his neck periodically for up to fifteen minutes separated by a small slightly moistened towel between the ice pack and Liam's skin. Liam leaves with his radiology script and returns in two days with x-rays of the lumbar spine and pelvis. These x-rays were taken on a 14" x 17" x-ray film and are large enough to reveal the lower spine, pelvis and upper portion of each leg bone or 'femur'. My measurements indicate that the left femur level is indeed 1/2 inch shorter than the right. Satisfied that we have a true leg length deficiency, I cast Liam's feet for the formulation of orthotics that will take approximately one week to formulate in a podiatric lab. The left orthotic will be raised 3/8's of an inch. (It would be difficult to use the lift if we gave him the full 1/2 inch as his orthotic would be so high that his heel might slip out of his left shoe. A 1/8-inch difference in leg length should be well tolerated and enable Liam to balance the head well enough to overcome his chronic neck stress.)

(It should be noted that the radiologist issuing the report makes no mention of the leg length discrepancy.)

Liam after Three Weeks of Orthotic Use

Liam has now been getting bi-weekly cervical adjustments and wearing his orthotics whenever he stands/walks. His last headache was a week and a half ago, milder and lasted only an hour. I'm happy with the improvement in the alignment of his atlas which is better positioned now following twelve spinal manipulations. I will continue to adjust Liam twice per week for two more weeks. If he continues to be headache free at that time he will be released. I advise Liam's mother to keep Liam in the orthotics and to see me in a year for a re-examination and a recasting of his feet for new orthotics as he grows. With time Liam's leg length may equalize but this is unlikely.

After two additional weeks of treatment and no more headaches, we say goodbye for now. A year later Liam has his follow-up; he had experienced no more headaches and is re-casted for new orthotics to match his larger feet.

Erin's Shin Splints

Erin, my oldest daughter of three, was a red-headed little cherub when her mother and I first realized at the age of about five months that her forefeet were turned in way too much. Forefoot adductus is not uncommon in children. Still in graduate school, I was lucky enough to find a smart young podiatrist who cast both her feet to correct the problem. At her young age, we were told she would need the casts for about eight weeks but should be able to make a full correction. The process was difficult for her two worried parents but Erin took it in the good-natured and happy style that was her hallmark and all turned out well.

At about nine years of age and perhaps seven years into my practice, Erin began to awake nightly with deep and severe shin pain often termed 'shin splints'. Her mother and I, arriving with aspirin and a glass of water, would rub her legs and put warm compresses on her shins. This would usually calm her pain and after an hour or so allow her to sleep. Taking a close look at my daughter I realized that she also had a marked leg length difference coupled with an inward rolling of her ankles and feet known as 'pronation'. This was coupled with a loss of the natural foot arch causing her to have 'flat feet' as well! How was it that I spent eight hours a day looking at patients and had never taken a good look at my own daughter! Now into my post-graduate orthopedic education, I was just learning to do castings for shoe orthotics but decided to bring Erin to a podiatrist well known in my town.

The day finally arrived a week later and my wife and I took daughter number one for her exam. Pointing out my observations, the podiatrist agreed that Erin needed orthotics to lessen her pronation, one of which would be elevated to compensate for the shorter leg. Back in the podiatrist office ten days later, Erin was fitted for her new orthotics. These we placed inside her shoes having removed the insoles that had come with them. Over the next few days, Erin's complaints of shin pain diminished. Within two weeks she was pain-free. Now, a mother herself, Erin continues to wear orthotics to correct her pronation and leg length difference remaining to this day. You can bet that I will be taking a close look at my grandchildren since body composition has a strong genetic link! Little Katie Rose and Jimmy Aiden could have their mother's short leg and pronated feet!

Childhood pain should never be overlooked. In cases similar to Erin's many doctors are quick to dismiss childhood complaints as growing pains. In my clinical opinion, there is no such thing as growing pains and normal childhood development should never be painful!

Helen's Vertigo

Sitting down to begin my office day, I check my emails and find the following message:

Hello, my name is Helen Maulder and I hope you can help me. I used to teach and drive and have a normal life until August of 2014 when I experienced an acute episode of pervasive dizziness. It has continued and my symptoms are so severe that I have been unable to work or drive for the past three years. I have been diagnosed with Meniere's Disease. I have fluctuating hearing loss, tinnitus, fullness/pressure in my ears and earaches. I have headaches and neck pain as well. The dizziness is the worst; my vertigo comes and goes but the pervasive dizziness/loss of balance is crippling. I went to a clinic for vestibular rehab for five months and felt best when they used the Saunder's Traction.

I was denied disability and do not receive social security benefits but I do receive food stamps. I am currently on Medicaid which does not cover chiropractic. I was able to be seen by a chiropractor last year who diagnosed me as having subluxations of my cervical vertebrae, possibly stemming from a motor vehicle whiplash some twenty years ago, but their fees were beyond my means. I had contacted one chiropractor who agreed to accept a nominal fee but he was located far from where I live. My only means of travel is by public transportation and the costs, even for a bus, I can't afford.

I now live in Greenwood Lake, New York, and was looking at your website. I can take the more inexpensive Dial-A-Bus over the mountain to Warwick and was hoping that you might consider seeing me at a reduced cost. All I want is to get my life back and to be able to drive and work again. I sit here as life passes me by and I am powerless to do anything about it. I believe chiropractic care could be helpful and I am hoping that you might be able to help me.

Thanks for reading this,
Helen Maulder

Cervical manipulation can be extremely effective at reducing vertigo, dizziness and tinnitus as is typified in a research study conducted in Switzerland in 2013. One hundred and seventy-seven adult patients with neck pain and dizziness began treatment consisting of chiropractic manipulation of the cervical spine. Outcome surveys conducted one, three and six months after beginning treatment demonstrated that 80% of the 177 patients with dizziness were significantly better with greatly decreased symptoms.[70]

A few days later Ms. Maulder, is sitting in my exam room with a sheaf of x-rays of the cervical spine newly performed at an area hospital. These I have ordered and her Medicaid has covered the cost even though they will not pay for chiropractic care. Although she had x-rays performed three years ago I feel these would be out of date as her cervical spine could have changed in the interim. Her new x-rays show moderate damage to the C5-C6 disc with thinning and some arthritic changes of the joints as well as a mild left shift of the atlas or uppermost vertebrae. Otherwise, her x-rays are quite unremarkable. (Lateral shifting of the atlas can affect balance, causing vertigo as the displacement places pressure on the brain stem which is housed within; a topic I'll cover later on in greater detail.)

Asking Helen to perform various balance maneuvers, some with her eyes closed, she nearly topples and has to reach to support herself on a nearby chair. Following several orthopedic tests to determine the status of the cervical spine and ruling out any contraindications to cervical manipulation we have a serious conversation. "Helen, you contacted me seeking chiropractic care and as you may know adjusting your cervical spine could be helpful in reducing your vertigo but I also want to advise you that there is a slight risk that the same manipulation could worsen your symptoms. In my opinion, if that were the case the effects would probably be of short duration but there is a very small chance that negative symptoms could be more prolonged."

Although negative risks are small this type of discussion is known as giving a patient an idea of potential harm to spinal manipulation and is considered important information so that a patient can make an informed choice about having their spine adjusted. (As you will have read, the risk of chiropractic intervention is a tiny fraction of that associated with medical intervention. A claim easily verified by looking at statistical outcome studies and malpractice insurance costs.)[71]

"Doctor Hargis, for the last three years I haven't been able to drive or work. If I want to leave my apartment I have to walk, take public transportation or call a friend. Do you have any idea what that's like? I am a prisoner to my vertigo and I need it to end! I want any help you can give me and I don't consider the risk high at all."

Getting the green light I proceed. Asking Helen to lie on her back upon a treatment table I deliver a fast tractive adjustment to correct her subluxated atlas. Following the adjustment I have Helen lie quietly for a few minutes. Upon arising she seems to be fine with no increase of vertigo and I ask her to return in two to three days. We continue the adjustments for three more visits at which time Helen reports a near-total reduction in her chronic vertigo and states she feels so well she has accepted an offer from her sister to join her in Florida to assist her in her real estate office! I warn her that she should continue the cervical spine adjustments as I am not satisfied that her atlas is yet entirely well positioned. She assures me she will continue with a new doctor in Florida if possible. While the patient's name was changed this is an accurate retailing of our encounter.

Judy's TMJ, Headaches and Forward Head Posture

Judy, now in her forties, is a busy bank manager, stressed to the max, with a three-year history of right-sided jaw pain and headaches. Her dentist has informed her that she is grinding her teeth at night and has made her a bite appliance that prevents her from damaging her teeth further but doesn't stop her clenching her jaw at night. She's bitten through two bite appliances in the past year!

After taking a careful history and examining her neck and posture I see that Judy carries her head far forward of its normal balance point which would be with the ear directly over the erect non-slumped shoulders. Forward head posture is the most common abnormality of the cervical spine and adversely affects the function of the TMJ. Forward head posture or FHP, retracts the position of the lower jaw stretching the joint capsule of the jaw and offsetting the proper fit and bite of the upper and lower teeth. This abnormal occlusion is stressing to the many muscles that move the jaw and will stress, tire and tighten the muscles of chewing or 'mastication'. FHP also stresses the TMJ joint, creating pain, inflammation and popping or grinding of the joint which over time can damage the joint cartilage and its bony surfaces.[72] Forward head posture also places tremendous strain on the structures of the spine and its supporting muscles and is a major cause of headaches.[73]

Forward Head Posture and the 48 Pound Head

The normal adult head weighs 10 to 12 pounds and for every inch we carry the head forward of its balance point the force needed to hold the head erect increases the heads weight by 100%[74] That means a 12-pound head carried three inches forward of its normal erect balanced posture now weighs 48 pounds! As we saw in the section discussing Sandra's condition this is akin to holding a bowling ball balanced above the elbow and slowly moving it forward. If we place the elbow on a support like a table and balance the ball directly above the elbow, this position requires little effort. However, as we move the ball forward and out of balance the muscles of our arm begin to strain and tire. The muscles acting to hold the head anchor into our rib cage and shoulder blades and insert into the vertebrae of the cervical spine and skull. Their fulcrum or lever of support is the spine itself and the increased force of holding the imbalanced head is generated directly through the delicate joints and discs of the neck. As you may imagine this will greatly accelerate the degeneration of the cervical spine! The March 2000 Mayo Clinic Health Letter, reported that prolonged FHP leads to increased "neck tension, disc herniations, arthritis and pinched nerves."

Forward head posture

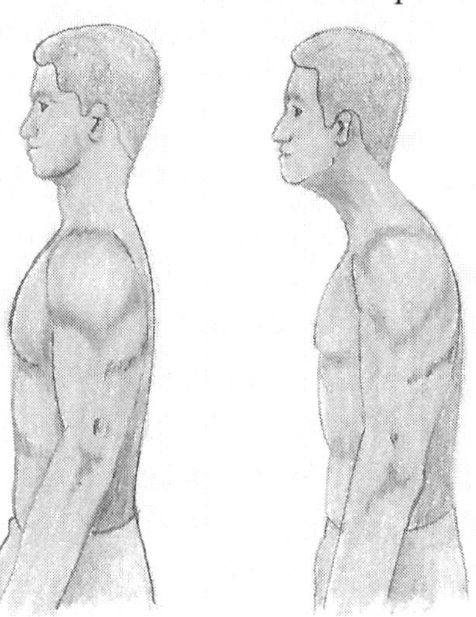

According to Rene Cailliet M.D., noted author, lecturer and former director of the department of physical medicine and rehabilitation at the University of Southern California, FHP not only magnifies the weight of the head but is capable of pulling the entire spine out of alignment and reducing vital lung capacity.[75] This impact on breathing is primarily due to inhibition of the muscles responsible for lifting the first rib during inhalation. Cailliet further states: "Most attempts to correct posture are directed toward the spine, shoulders and pelvis. All are important, but head position takes precedence over all others. The body follows the head. Therefore, the entire body is best aligned by first restoring proper functional alignment to the head".

Dr. Roger Sperry, Nobel Prize Recipient for Brain Research, demonstrated that 90% of the brain's energy output is used in relating the physical body to gravity. Only 10% has to do with thinking, metabolism, and healing. Consequently, FHP will cause the brain to rob energy from thinking, metabolism and immune function to deal with abnormal gravity/posture relationships and processing.[76]

Degenerative neck pain goes hand-in-hand with balance problems especially in the elderly. Degeneration damages and diminishes sensitive balance receptors located throughout the cervical spine and paraspinal muscles that govern ones balance. FHP and degeneration of the neck cause alteration in the ear blood-flow circulation that leads to hearing loss, vertigo and tinnitus.

The brainstem is the posterior part of the brain adjoining and structurally continuous with the spinal cord. The lower aspect of the brainstem is housed inside the upper two cervical vertebrae known as the atlas and axis.[78] Though small, this is an extremely important part of the brain as neural control of many complex body functions begin and end in the brainstem. The brainstem provides the main motor and sensory innervations to the face and neck via the cranial nerves, ten of which begin here. Brainstem irritation can affect motor control of our muscles, our sense of vibration and proprioception (sense of body position, gravity and pressure) as well as our perception of pain, temperature, itch, and touch. The brainstem also plays an important role in the regulation of our heart rate, breathing, sleep and appetite.[79] It's interesting to conjecture just what effects major stress on the atlas and axis vertebrae might have when excessive load from forward head position distorts their movement patterns and stretches the brainstem itself! More will be said about this later.

Back to Judy

Asking Judy to lie down face upward on a treatment table I palpate the muscles in Judy's neck and jaw. Both areas are tight and inflamed from the constant stress of her head position. I let her know that her spinal vertebrae, subjected to this prolonged stress, need to be manipulated to increase flexibility and normal movement patterns to the cervical spine. In this case, some light massage to the neck followed by my spinal manipulation is indicated as Judy gives her permission for the latter. Palpating the jaw I explain the need for deeper 'trigger point' pressure here to release some of the deep tension in the muscles of chewing or 'mastication'. These muscles, four in number, are the lateral and internal pterygoids, masseter and temporalis. Judy's masseter (lower outer jaw muscle), is especially tight and I ask her to stretch the jaw wide as I apply a moderate downward force to her chin with my left thumb while using my right thumb to goad her right masseter just atop the jaw joint proper. This is done with deep pressure for about 15 seconds. Asking Judy to sit, she immediately feels a lessening of jaw pain as the deep tension in the muscles has been released somewhat by the trigger point therapy.

Although less common than muscle strain, there are many legitimate cases where the muscles are so fatigued and overworked that they will become tight and spastic. Long-standing stress without acute injury is usually the culprit. Although there had been no 'injury' to Judy's jaw the chronic effect of having an imbalanced bite due to her FHP had badly affected the muscles of the jaw producing spasm. Direct trigger point therapy releases the jaw spasm with an immediate reduction in jaw pain and improved bite motion and width. However, caution must be observed in validating this as deep muscle goading is injurious to soft tissue strains and tears.

Following her treatment which includes ultrasound therapy to the jaw and neck, I send her for x-rays of the cervical spine. Returning the following day, x-rays of the cervical spine indicate the early onset of spinal degeneration with narrowing of the spinal discs and some arthritic changes to the spinal joints. In addition to manipulation of the cervical spine and ultrasound therapy to the neck and jaw, she will be given exercises for the upper back and shoulders to bring them into better alignment/posture. These will include resistance band exercises for the back and 'Neck Correct/Curve Restorer' exercises to reduce the FHP.

Judy is told to sleep on her back as side and stomach sleeping stress the jaw and neck and to use ice packs at home in both areas. I also instruct her to begin chewing gum. This is a tactic to make her aware of her jaw and to interrupt and lessen the jaw clenching.

Judy Week Four

Judy is doing better and regular treatments have reduced both her jaw, neck and headache complaints quite a bit. She'll begin the exercise regimen and we'll follow-up with comparison x-rays of the C spine (cervical spine) in six months to monitor her progress with the Neck Correct as she improves her neck posture. (The Neck Correct will be discussed later under the section dedicated to 'Forward Head Posture').

Visit HealingTheHumanMachine.com for a video demonstrating the Neck Correct or to order one.

Peter's TFL

Peter accompanies his wife Janet to my office on most occasions and sits quietly in my waiting room. I've been treating Janet now for some weeks and she is responding well. Following her visit this morning she asks if I could help her husband with his lateral leg pain. She explains that for the past four years Peter has experienced chronic right lateral leg pain with a year of physical therapy and consultations with an orthopedist and pain specialist to no avail. So I ask her to call Peter from the waiting room and bring him in.

"Pete is stubborn. I don't think he'll come."

So I go out to the waiting room and ask Pete to come with me. "So Pete, I understand you're having a leg problem."

Pete looks at his wife of twenty-something years. I'm hoping they won't need a marriage counselor after this conversation. "I am and have for the past four years! I also have back pain."

Peter gives me a fuller picture of his past medical care and relates that an MRI of his lower back taken at the start of his complaints revealed multiple disc protrusions and the doctors have stated that his leg pain is due to his spinal pathology. Examining his deep tendon reflexes, all of which are normal for the lower extremities, I ask him to perform a Dejerine's maneuver which is an orthopedic/chiropractic test to indicate disc compression of the spinal cord or spinal nerve roots. While Pete is sitting I ask him to take a deep breath, holding in the air and to then strain downward as if he were attempting to move his bowels for ten seconds. During this time he is placing a constant downward abdominal pressure which will magnify the force of any disc compression on the spinal cord or spinal nerves increasing leg or back pain. In Peter's case, the test elicits no pain. Asking him to lie on the non-painful side I place a pillow between his legs and begin to palpate the painful area of his lateral right leg from the hip downward to the knee with my fingers. Moderate pressure to several areas from the hip to the knee brings on a strong avoidance response from Pete.

"Peter, have you ever had pain below the knee or numbness in the foot?

"No, I haven't."

"How did you do with the physical therapy, the orthopedist and pain specialist?"

"Well, I went on and off for a year to PT. Sometimes when I left I would feel a little better and at other times I could barely walk out of there. They gave me one stretch to do for the lateral leg and it laid me up in bed for a week after! The orthopedist said my leg pain was due to my back but the discs were not so bad as to need surgery and the pain specialist gives me meds which I don't normally take because they make me feel drugged-up and lousy."

"Do you still do stretches?"

"Sometimes I do and vary the type a bit but it doesn't seem to help much."

I explain the analog pain scale and ask Peter to rate his pain.

"On a good day a three and on a bad day a seven."

"Pete, I want you to bring in the MRI of your back. There's no indication that your leg pain is related to your low back, in fact, I think you're dealing with two separate and distinct issues; low back pain and a TFL injury." TFL stands for tensor fasciae latae. The TFL is a combination of muscles and fascia running from the hip and buttock down to the knee on the outer side of the leg. Injury to these tissues is common and usually brought on by limping or other irregularities of gait or by direct injury."

"My doctors said I had TFL but that it was related to the back. Doc let me show you something." Peter brings my attention to a nodule about the size of a small egg just below the surface of the skin, in the lateral/anterior thigh."

"When did you get this?"

"About four years ago when the pain started. I was splitting wood and tripped over a piece in the grass."

"And you didn't think that might not be connected to your leg pain?"

"Well I did but the doctors ordered the MRI and had a different opinion."

"Peter that nodule is scar tissue in the muscle, probably from injury experienced in the fall. The multiple tender points throughout your lateral leg and the absence of any numbness or reflex changes of your legs makes it unlikely we're dealing with a disc pathology affecting your leg. I think you have a good 'old fashioned' blunt trauma injury to the lateral leg coupled with back strain that's unrelated to your discs and I'm going to hold to that opinion until I see your MRI. In the meantime, if you're willing, we'll begin some therapy that I think will be helpful. So please, no more sleeping on the right side, no stretching, rubbing the leg, no heat only ice packs at home and ultrasound here in the office. Oh, and I want you to be careful how you walk with no limping. When you walk you need to smoothly transition your weight from side to side."

Pete's Second Visit Two Days Later

"How's the Leg?"

"No difference yet."

"It's too early. It will take a few days for the swelling to start to go down. We'll just keep doing the right therapy and things should start to go our way pretty soon." I pull up the MRI Pete has provided, seeing that while Pete has multiple disc protrusions in the lumbar spine they are relatively small. None are capable of compressing the spinal cord or spinal nerves. This further solidifies the diagnosis of a stand-alone back strain and a TFL injury which hasn't healed. Therapy continues.

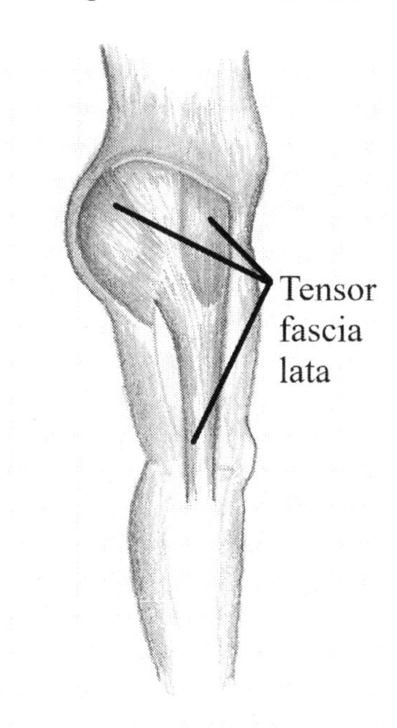

Pete at Four Months

Pete's care has been quite frequent, (3 times per week), receiving ultrasound and ice pack applications to his back and leg now for four months. About two and a half months in we began rehab exercises. He now had no leg pain and rates his back pain as a 1 or 2 on a bad day and 0 usually. Pete was kind enough to give me a nice review many of which can be found at Warwick Brain and Spine Therapy.

"After enduring back pain for 4 years, I have finally gotten relief by going to Dr Hargis. I went to an orthopedic surgeon, physical therapy, a spine specialist and a pain management doctor and not one of them helped my pain. My wife, who is a patient of Dr Hargis, suggested that he might be able to help me. After reading my x-rays and MRI, he came up with a treatment plan of adjustments and ultrasound therapy. Now I am nearly pain free, having no pain at all on many days." Peter S.

Visit HealingTheHumanMachine.com for a video discussing

TFL syndrome.

Maggie's Constipation, Rectal Pain and Degenerated Lumbar Spine

When I first saw Maggie she was truly in a pitiful state. Age seventy, she had severe low back pain, constipation and constant rectal pain that had plagued her for years. Having gone through two surgeries intended to provide her relief, her condition had worsened. The first surgery, a hysterectomy, was performed to remove a small benign mass that was thought to be pressing on her colon, causing her constipation; the second surgery to correct a rectocele or out-pouching of the rectal pathway. Following each, she experienced increased constipation with more bowel meds and antidepressants. She had come to me because she had exhausted every other avenue of treatment.

During her exam, it was noted that she had a short leg, (common to low back pain patients) and scoliosis. Further, her pelvic joints were locked upon 'motion palpation', (a method of examination employed by chiropractors to check for good spinal and pelvic mobility). Smooth movement and glide of the large pelvic bones in their attachment to the central sacral bone is expected but Maggie's pelvic motion was extremely limited, almost solidly fixed indicating pelvic subluxation. Arriving for her second visit with the standing x-rays I had ordered, it was observed that she had a right short leg of approximately 3/4 of an inch, resulting in a scoliosis or right sided spinal curvature. She also had substantial degeneration of the spinal discs in her lower back from the years of walking and lifting out of balance. Since the lumbar nerves supply the colon and rectum, degeneration of the lumbar spinal discs had likely resulted in reduced nerve flow from the spine to the colon and presented a reasonable explanation for her difficult bowel movements. It was interesting to note that Maggie was unaware of her leg length difference which was plainly evident on her standing x-rays and previously undiagnosed. The reading radiologist report of the x-rays I had requested did not mention the leg length difference.

Formulating podiatric grade shoe orthotics with a right 1/2 inch lift, I began over the next few weeks to begin the slow and gentle process of low back stretch and manipulation to unlock her pelvic structures and to increase spinal and pelvic motion that had eroded over her seventy years. Each series of spinal adjustments and stretch treatments gave her increasing mobility to the spine and pelvis resulting in better neural communication to her digestive tract. Simultaneously I advised her to throw the laxatives in the trash and begin a regimen of fruit and vegetable smoothies twice per day accompanied by more water intake. Within two weeks, her bowels were beginning to move with greater ease and her spinal pain and motion had improved substantially. Following three months of therapy, Maggie greatly improved. Now I treat Maggie once weekly; her Medicare pays for her visits. She is nearly pain-free and everything is moving along nicely!

Susan's Carpal Tunnel

Susan a 24-year-old graduate student is describing her carpal tunnel pain while she constantly massages and squeezes both her right wrist and forearm. Ongoing for six months now and getting much worse Susan consulted with an orthopedic surgeon who has diagnosed her condition as carpal tunnel syndrome (CTS) and is recommending a surgical release of the area by cutting the transverse carpal ligament of the wrist. This thin membrane covers the delicate median nerve and attaches to the carpal or wrist bones creating a narrow canal that houses the median nerve.

While some patients are recommended to have steroid injections for the carpal tunnel prior to surgery this has been shown to be ineffective. In a study by Dr. D.E. Hoffman, he concludes, "Significant symptom relief beyond one month has not been demonstrated. Two local corticosteroid injections do not provide a significant added clinical benefit compared to one injection."[80] In another study by Dr. A.C. Hui and colleagues, the authors conducted a trial of fifty patients with carpal tunnel syndrome (CTS), where 25 had surgery and 25 had steroid injections only. At twenty weeks the participants rated their improvement on a 0 (no improvement) to 50 (best result) scale. The steroid group rated their improvement at 8.7 (poor). Most interesting, the surgical group only rated their improvement at 24.2 out of a possible 50![81]

Statistics indicate that at least one in four patients do not fare well with carpal tunnel surgery although every year more than 500,000 American's receive this procedure. Treatment failure and complication rates of CTS surgery and other forms of treatment vary greatly with mixed results. Complications after surgery may include nerve damage with tingling, numbness, infection, scarring, pain and stiffness of the wrist or hand. Loss of wrist strength is a complication that affects up to a third of patients. Some patients who have jobs requiring significant strength of the hand and wrist can no longer perform their duties. These patients may also have problems in other parts of the upper body, including elbows and shoulders. Studies indicate that 10-15% of patients change jobs after a CTS operation.

CTS is hallmarked by pain, numbness and tingling, in the part of the hand that receives sensation from the median nerve. The main symptom of CTS is intermittent numbness of the thumb, index and middle fingers and the radial (thumb) side of the ring finger. The numbness often occurs at night due to sleep positions that stress or compress the inner wrist such as the wrists being held flexed during sleep or sleeping on one's side with the hand and wrist under the pillow and head. Pain may also extend up the arm leading to discomfort extending to the forearm, elbow and shoulder. Long-standing carpal tunnel syndrome may lead to permanent nerve damage with constant numbness and atrophy of some of the muscles of the hand.

While carpal tunnel symptoms may result from an injury that causes internal scarring or misaligned wrist bones, the use of vibrating tools or manual labor, today more and more people are incurring CTS due to the repetitive nature of keyboarding and computer use. Computer use has exploded with many individuals spending hours per day at work or at home keyboarding, socializing, perusing the internet and playing games. Contact on the delicate inner wrist is common with computing and even though we may use soft pads under the wrist areas to ease discomfort these soft pads continue to over-pressurize the carpal tunnel.[82] Over time the area becomes more and more inflamed and irritated.

In Susan's case, she adds more injury to the area as she constantly squeezes her painful wrist and forearm attempting to mediate the pain and I explain all this to her.

"Susan, how did this all get started?"

"I was writing a research paper and spending long hours on the computer when I began to notice some mild numbness in my right hand."

"Anything else?"

"I was working at a homeless shelter on the weekends serving and preparing food."

"Do you still volunteer?"

"No, I can't hold the spoons and knives anymore. My hand is

too numb."

"What have you done to relieve the pain?"

"Well I take aspirin which helps for a while and I got a jelly pad to go under my wrist when I keyboard. I also do some exercises I found recommended on the Internet. I have a brace I wear sometimes during the day and at night. Do you want to see it?" She reaches down to her pocketbook and pulls out a carpal wrist brace.

"Would you put that on."

She does so and I note the underside of the brace lies snugly against the carpal region and that the metal bar incorporated into the palm side of the brace bends her hand backward slightly.

"Would you take off the brace now and show me the exercises."

Susan places both palms together stretching her wrists deeply at right angles to the palm. These maneuvers are routinely recommended by M.D.'s and P.T.'s and in my experience do nothing more than further irritate the median nerve.

"I also squeeze a soft sponge-like ball."

"Sue, the median nerve is extremely delicate and can be easily bruised or irritated to the point that the nerve and the carpal area become highly swollen. Once this is the case steps should be taken to reduce pressure and swelling in the area. Contrary to what you've been told, stretches narrow the carpal tunnel and squeeze the median nerve producing more irritation. I'd like you to stop the exercises and no more squeezing the arms and wrists; squeezing feels good for the moment because it interrupts pain sensations to the brain but only irritates the area more."

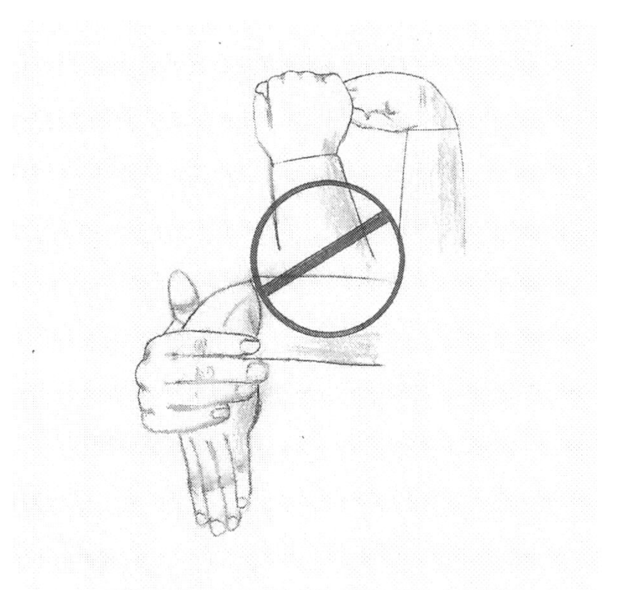

Carpal tunnel stretches to avoid

"What about my 'jelly pad' I use when keyboarding?"

"Have you heard of Isaac Newton's third law? No? Newton was a scientist and found that for every action, there is an equal and opposite reaction. Another way of putting it is that for every force you exert there is an equal and opposite force pushing back on you. Even though your jelly pad is soft it's still pressing into the delicate inner wrist and median nerve with the weight of your forearm and hand upon it. That's about three to five pounds of force. What I would like, is that when you keyboard, find a way to rest the upper forearms keeping the wrists out of contact with hard or soft surfaces. Perhaps you can elevate your arms and wrists away from any contact with surfaces when using a computer. Raising your chair may help as well."

"Also the wrist braces you're using should not place your wrists in a flexed backward position and the metal bar shouldn't be applying any pressure to the inner wrist. I'd like you to avoid crafting or other endeavors that will overwork the wrists until we have this well under control. We'll begin therapy with ultrasound in a water bath three times per week and you can apply ice packs 'lightly' to the wrist, time permitting, every hour or so for 15 minutes.

With treatment, we should see a nice reduction of your symptoms within the next three weeks." I also recommend curcumin and give her instructions for its use which is covered in detail later on.

Conservative methods of treatment for CTS were evaluated looking at 33 trials conducted by research groups between 1985 and 2006. The different treatment methods studied were injections, oral therapies, physical therapies, therapeutic exercises and splints. Interestingly the studies indicated that ultrasound therapy was effective in treating CTS and that exercise therapy was not![83]

Ultrasound is a sound wave therapy and like sonar can be transmitted through water into a body part. This is especially useful if the body part is irregular in contour or very delicate as is the case of the carpal tunnel and median nerve. Most carpal tunnel syndromes can be healed conservatively without surgery by strict compliance with the methods described here.

It should be noted that the median nerve emerges between the vertebrae of the cervical spine and travels through the shoulder and elbow before reaching the hand. Compression or pathology at any of these locations can affect the nerve. With Susan, these areas were examined and found to be normal and not impacting her wrist complaint.

Susan Week Four

Susan has now received 9 ultrasound therapy sessions in our office and has avoided pressuring or compressing maneuvers and postures to the carpal tunnel region along with frequent ice pack applications for three weeks. Her pain/numbness score was an 8 and now is a 3. She is on the right track and we will continue the same therapy and should see a complete resolution of her carpal tunnel issues.

(Later on we will discuss the 'Carpal Shield' carpal tunnel brace, which later came to be, and would have been used to more quickly end her discomfort if available at the time.)

Visit HealingTheHumanMachine.com for a video discussing proper carpal tunnel care.

Charlie's Bilateral Carpal Tunnel and the Evolution of the 'Carpal Shield' Carpal Tunnel Device

Charlie is ten years old and quite a rarity. Carpal tunnel syndrome (CTS) is most uncommon in children, (it's becoming more prevalent with increased computer use) and Charlie has carpal tunnel in both hands! Whenever he writes or keyboards his hands go numb especially in the wrist, palm and thumb to middle finger. Now he is even waking up due to numbness and hand pain at night. Mrs. Hinds, Charlie's mom, has taken him now to two hand surgeons and both have suggested bilateral carpal tunnel surgery. This procedure requires cutting the transverse carpal ligament passing over the median nerve and forming the 'roof' of the carpal tunnel. By cutting this retaining ligament median nerve pressure is usually released. CT surgery is no 'cakewalk' however and about a quarter or more of these procedures lead to long term problems like scarring, more pain, more numbness, loss of grip strength and additional (often unsuccessful) surgeries. Most people wouldn't think of consulting a chiropractor for carpal tunnel, even one with an orthopedic specialty, but Mrs. Hinds is desperate and I've helped her out in the past.

Putting Charlie through some basic maneuvers I see that flexion of the wrist and my light finger pressure into the carpal tunnel area quickly brings on Charlie's hand and finger numbness; a classic sign of the disorder.

"Charlie, what do you like to do? What are your hobbies?"

"Well, I like to play games on the computer."

Mom laughs, "Charlie's only hobby is sitting in front of his computer for hours a day."

"And how do you rest your hands while you're on your computer?"

They both pause and Charlie says, "On my desk?"

"How long have you been into the computers so heavily and when did the numbness start?"

"I got my computer a year ago and..."

"Charlie's been having problems with his hands for about six months," says mom. "Could that have something to do with the problem?"

"Well let's see; how are your hands feeling right this moment Charlie?"

"They're not too numb now."

"Okay. Charlie, come over to this counter and place both of your palms and wrists flat on the surface."

Charlie does so and about twenty seconds later states, "My hands are getting numb!"

"Okay, so just leave them there for a minute."

Fifteen seconds later Charlie says, "Really numb."

"Okay, that's enough. Charlie, come and sit on my exam table. Charlie does and I examine his neck for spinal alignment. Nerves from the cervical vertebrae innervate the hand and contribute several nerve branches that form the median nerve before it passes down through the arm and wrist. Misalignment of the cervical vertebrae can pressure and inflame these nerves leading from the spine to magnify/exacerbate carpal tunnel syndrome. If any misalignment of the C spine were found spinal manipulation would be indicated. Palpation indicates the vertebrae are well aligned.

"Mrs. Hinds, Charlie, I think I've found the problem. Your constant computer use is placing too much pressure on the carpal tunnel area. You're going to have to limit your time there. Try to stay totally away from the computer for two weeks."

Charlie looks stunned and turns to his mother pleading for intervention.

Mom looks just as upset and says, "Isn't there any other way? Charlie loves his games and he plays with friends. How about using one of those soft things, those cushions or 'jelly pads' under the wrist?"

"They are soft but create the same pressure. Charlie's hand, wrist and forearm weigh roughly three pounds so that weight is pushing into the carpal region even resting on a soft pad."

Charlie is now tearing up and Mom is beside herself. As I sit quietly for a few moments and think about the problem. "Tell you what, I have an idea: I can make molds of Charlie's hands and cast plastic guards he can wear to protect the carpal area so that there is no pressure on the inner wrist when he keyboards. It will take me two to three weeks to have them ready. They'll also be expensive because it will require several hours of my time."

"How expensive and will they work?"

"I believe it will work. As to the cost;" I try to calculate the time involved with making the plaster casts, carving a protective dome into the casts and vacuum molding plastic sheets into the proper shape, trimming out the casts and affixing a strap to each appliance as he will need one for each hand. These thoughts are moderated by the fact that I like a challenge, I've never tried this before and I want to keep it affordable. "Six hundred dollars. Sound fair?"

"If it fixes the problem and prevents the need for surgery it will be a bargain!", says Charlie's mother.

(I wish I had asked for more money.)

Asking Charlie and his mom to come back in two days, I mix enough plaster to make two molds of Charlie's right and left hand/wrist and lower forearm. I mix up a moderate pile of soft plaster and lower each hand, in turn, downward into the plaster in a keyboarding position. These molds when dry will replicate Charlie's keyboarding hand position and the contours of his palm/wrist and forearm. These negative plaster casts I will then carve to create a depression at the carpal area. When the heat-moldable plastic is vacuumed down into the carved molds a slim plastic shield will have been created that comfortably fits the contours of each of Charlie's hands and the raised dome will ensure Charlie places no pressure on the CT while keyboarding. At least that's the plan.

(I was lucky to find a place nearby that sold me a vacuum mold machine and it only cost me $1100 bucks! It was money well spent as you will soon learn.)

Two Weeks Later and Charlie Returns

Charlie's carpal braces are now ready. They are thin semi-rigid plastic 'shields' that cup the meaty part of Charlie's palm and upper wrist above the carpal tunnel area. A strap is attached, similar to a buckle watchband, to secure the braces into position. The cool thing about the shields is the raised dome over the carpal tunnel region allowing no pressure to pass through to the area! As the wearer keyboards, the weight of the resting hand is transferred to the palm and upper wrist.

Sending Charlie home I ask Mrs. Hinds to report back in three weeks and sternly instruct Charlie not to keyboard without them. Just two weeks later Mrs. Hinds is on the phone to report that Charlie has been using the carpal shields daily and has no more tingling or numbness in his hands. As I think about the result I realize the potential for the widespread use of such a device.

The Carpal Shield

The Carpal Shield is unique, featuring a light, comfortable and non-restrictive design allowing free use of the hand when worn. The raised dome directly over the carpal tunnel region allows for no compression to the delicate nerves of the inner wrist while keyboarding, performing general office duties or while sleeping with your hand under your pillow.

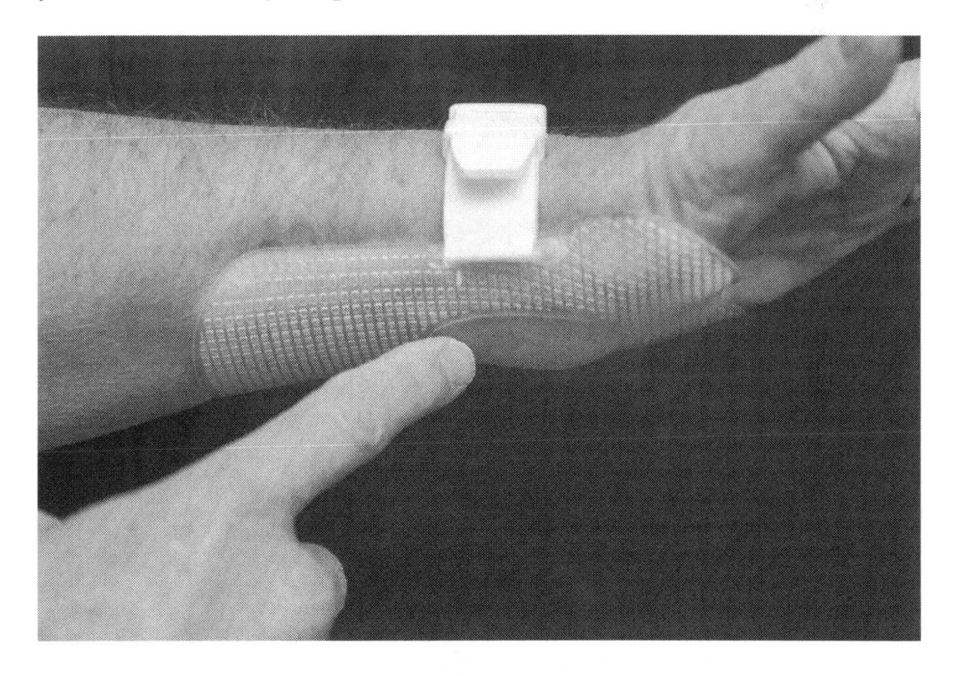

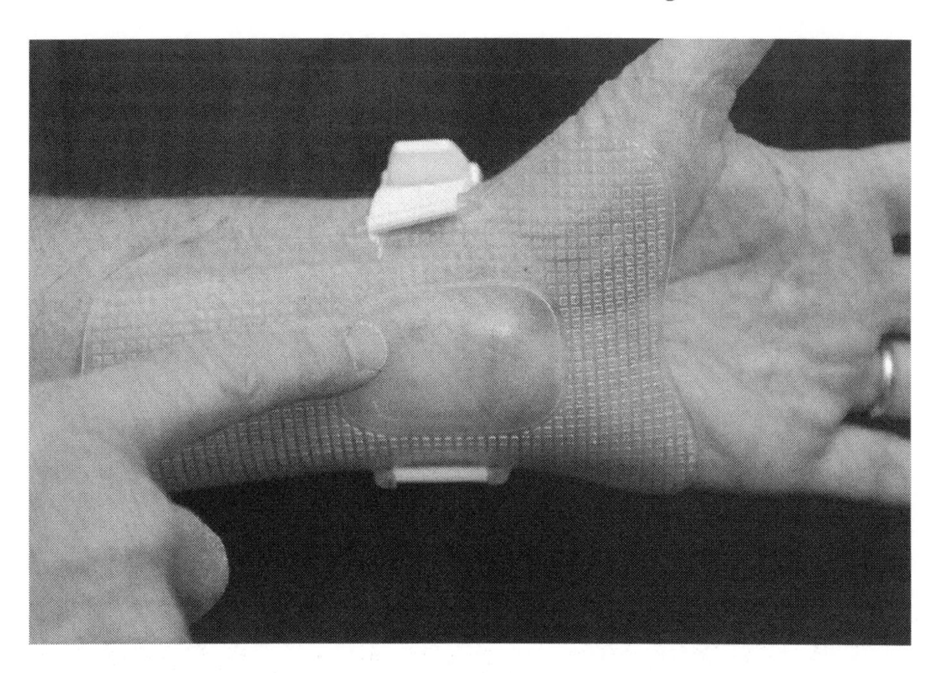

Currently under development, the 'Carpal Shield' is patented and should be available to the public in the next few months. Among various retail outlets, the device will likely be sold on Amazon as well. The cost of the 'Carpal Shield' when in full production, should be in the range of forty to fifty dollars or so and will be a definite boon to the treatment of carpal tunnel syndrome hopefully preventing countless surgeries. Prior to full production we are providing custom 3D printed braces for those with severe carpal tunnel pain or those considering surgery. Custom prints are available at a slightly greater cost and wait time of two to three weeks.

Visit HealingTheHumanMachine.com for a video demonstrating the Carpal Shield or to order one in your size and hand, either custom printed of after full production.

John's Calf Pain

John a local school administrator is an avid tennis player. This past summer he played a tiring tennis match with a buddy. As he was leaving the courts he meets a friend who had been stood up by his match partner and so kindly agreed to also play the friend in a second grueling match. Afterward, thoroughly exhausted, he returns home to soak in his hot tub. He feels a little better afterward but his calves are somewhat sore. Waking the next morning he barely makes it to the bathroom so painful are his calf muscles. The following day he is no better and sees his physician who prescribes ibuprofen and muscle relaxants while suggesting mild stretch and hot packs.

After two weeks with no relief, his doctor orders a Doppler study for blood clots and finding none sends him for PT. Physical therapy consists of stretching and strengthening exercises for the calves and legs coupled with massage. He completes only a few sessions as each therapy session leaves him in more pain. Fully six months later at our weekly Rotary club meeting, I ask him about his tennis game. He informs me he hasn't been playing much as any physical activity significantly increases his leg pain, which then flares for several days afterward. Massage, stretch and warm baths ease the pain for a while. During the meeting, he makes an appointment to see me asking if I have any advice in the meantime. I tell him to stop any sports activity as well as any stretch, massage and heat and to start applying ice packs instead.

When he comes into the office nearly a week later he had a big smile on his face. "You're not going to believe this but I already feel a little better."

"Did you begin following my advice on day one?"

"I did!"

"You should be feeling better. It's been five days."

"Can it start to change that quickly?"

"You bet; as long as you do all the right things, are relatively healthy, eat right, take it easy, use the right therapy and don't smoke;

(smoking delays healing significantly.) Most inflammatory processes will continue to swell for two to three days after you stop stressing and re-injuring the area as up to that point you've been doing everything wrong. After that swelling should begin to dissipate and the pain should begin to naturally decrease."

Examining the painful calves I first note that no substantial redness or heat is emanating from the calves, a sign that might indicate a blood clot or infection, (although it would be extremely unlikely that both calves would be involved at the same time or that a clot or infection would be present if the patient were improved as was John on this visit). With the same pressure I might squeeze a lemon to check for ripeness, I now press into the calf area of each leg noting John's complaints of soreness and his reaction to draw away from my pressure. Interestingly he can lift his heels while standing without much pain but pushing on his forefoot to stretch the foot toward his knee produces pain in the belly of each calf indicating tissue damage.

"John we can safely begin ultrasound therapy and ice pack applications. I would like you to continue to ice for 15 minutes every hour or two throughout the day when you have the time and do absolutely no stretch, massage or extended walking. Also if you use a recliner I want you to avoid allowing your calves to rest on the raised foot portion. This can exert undue pressure on the calves and keep them bruised. You may be able to place a pillow under the knees in such a fashion as to avoid this pressure or avoid the reclining position altogether. We'll do three ultrasound sessions per week for three to four weeks and by that time you should be healed enough to start rehab exercises."

John's Calf Pain, Week Four, Rehab Time

John has now improved a lot and has minimal calf pain rated at 2 on the analog scale. John is now instructed to do 10 heel lifts in the morning and 10 lifts in the evening beginning from a neutral standing position. He is to do them slowly with no bouncing and cannot do them from a step as at no time do we want the heel to drop below the plane of the foot which would introduce a stretch to the exercise for which John is not ready. Following two weeks of exercise in this fashion and working up to twenty heel raises twice per day over this period he can begin a walking program over level terrain. Slowly week by week he can increase the incline of his walks to provide more calf stretch motion to his gait. This can be done on a treadmill at a slow to moderate pace if the treadmill deck is firm and not bouncy. During this process, it is advisable to continue his ultrasound therapy as this will ensure more and better physiological repair of the calf tissue lessening the chance of redundant scar tissue formation. The bottom line: take it slow and use common sense in rehab.

"Can I start playing tennis again?"

"Your legs won't be ready for quick transitional movements needed for a vigorous tennis match for about two to three months but you can do some slower movements and ball strikes to maintain your hand/eye coordination. I recommend a racquetball court for that or tennis ball machine, just solo, no opponents.

Mabel's Hip Pain

Hip pain can result from a degenerated hip but is more commonly a muscular condition in my experience and either can be felt as being anyplace from mid buttock to upper leg or even the front of the pelvis. True hip pain is generated from the hip socket or 'acetabulum' and the joining of the ball-like 'head' of the upper leg bone or 'femur'. A weight-bearing (standing) x-ray of the hip easily demonstrates the thickness of hip cartilage. A quarter-inch space between the top of the femur and the hip socket is normal and less space indicates diminished cartilage thickness associated with wear. If there is no or little space (cartilage) revealed on the x-ray and the bone of the femur head is near to or in contact with the bone of the acetabulum or hip socket then you likely have pain relating to a degenerative hip and surgery is typically indicated if sufficiently severe. However, many muscles and tendons attach to the hip and it is far more common to have hip pain as a result of strain/injury to the soft tissue structures.

Mabel enters the exam room limping and holding her hand on her right buttock. She says she has been experiencing hip pain in the same area for a month with sudden onset following a camping trip and some 'vigorous' firewood collecting. Since a degenerated hip usually has a slow onset over months or years with slowly increasing pain a sudden onset would indicate more of a soft tissue problem. Fortunately, Mable has the forethought to come with x-rays of the low back and hip as she is treating with her local MD who has ordered the studies and advised a heating pad and stretches. The x-rays show good separation between the femur head and hip socket but digital examination reveals muscular swelling and tenderness in the mid-right buttock. Asking Mable to lie on her left side and then stomach, I ask her to lift her right leg against my resistance which provokes her pain which is centered in the musculature of her buttock and upper leg. Mable has no leg pain or numbness below the knee so sciatic pain is ruled out. My diagnosis is of a soft tissue strain/tear with inflammation. Her x-rays also demonstrate rotational malposition of the lumbar vertebrae which have been stressed by her chronic limp. I explain this as well and the need for some lumbar spine adjustments.

Maple had been shown stretches by her MD and was performing them daily including back and leg twists and pulling her right knee to her chest. As we have seen, stretching soft tissue injuries is akin to pouring gasoline on a flame!

"No more stretches Mable and do not lie on your right side in bed. Also no propping up in bed with pillows to watch TV or read. No heat and no tub baths which stretch the lower back. Also along with discontinuing the stretching please don't cross your right leg over your left as this stretches the hip as well." (I also explain the need for a smooth gait without limping and the need for regular icing at home.

"I have a massage scheduled for tomorrow. Should I go."

"Any amount of physical stress in the area will prevent healing. This includes stretch, massage, vibration and heat. Also, you need to be here regularly for ultrasound (US) and frequently use ice packs at home." We discuss all of these topics in detail along with her x-ray study.

Two weeks and six treatments latter, consisting of spinal manipulation, ultrasound and ice packs, Mable is out of pain.

Out of Pain and Out of Here! Mable feels well!

"Doc I feel great. I don't think I need to come anymore."

"Mable, the absence of pain means the swelling has subsided however the area is fragile and will be healing for several weeks or months. I suggest you continue to receive your therapy three times a week for three to four more weeks at a minimum while you continue to follow all the rules of posture. This will allow for better healing and decrease the chances of re-occurrence and scar tissue formation."

While nearly everyone equates the absence of pain with wellness this is a big mistake! Soft tissue inflammation creates pain and is directly proportional to it. Tissue inflammation and pain depart early in the process of healing and well before its completion. The very delicate and randomized tissue patch or intramuscular 'scab' is just beginning to change its structure toward more normal tissue when swelling and pain have dissipated. Mistaking the absence of pain as a sign of complete healing of a muscle or other soft tissue tear and getting right back into a demanding lifestyle is the biggest reason for re-injury. This can also lead to possible scaring, weak tissue repair and chronic pain. When pain is gone ultrasound is still indicated for several weeks. This will ensure the best healing as the sound waves generated from US therapy improve the structural remodeling of healing tissue.

Additionally, spinal vertebrae out of position are seldom put right with one or two adjustments. Aligning the spine properly often takes weeks or months of care but the benefits can be life-changing.

Nick's Elbow Pain

Nick makes the best pizza. Sitting down to a particularly pleasing slice of spicy pepperoni Nick comes over and we 'shoot the breeze'. I notice Nick is wearing a support brace around the right elbow. "What's up with the elbow, Nick"

"I don't know doc but the dammed thing is killing me for the past few weeks."

He goes on to say that for the past six months he has had a sore elbow and at a recent visit to an area orthopedist, he was x-rayed and told that he may need surgery as the elbow is arthritic. Nick has been attending PT but after five visits he seems to be making little progress. Nick is concerned that he may not be able to continue the physical nature of his work. I see as I'm getting this information, that Nick is massaging his right elbow with his left thumb.

"Can you do anything Doc?

Later that week Nick is sitting in my exam room and I'm looking at his x-ray films. He does have arthritic changes of the elbow but the degenerative changes seem mild to moderate in nature and there is still adequate space between bony structures.

"Nick, how do you sleep?"

"I used to sleep on my stomach but that hurts the elbow so now I try to stay on my back or left side with a pillow under my right arm. It makes my elbow feel better." Sleeping with the arm above the head or under the pillow introduces stretch and rotation to the elbow which will exacerbate elbow pain.

"Good. Did you ever injure the elbow?"

"Not really. I pitched baseball in high school and had a little pain now and then but no big deal."

"How long have you been making pizzas?"

Nick laughs, "A long time. Maybe longer than you been walking."

As Nick is giving me his history he once again begins to rub the elbow.

"Okay, I want you to make a fist and give me some slight resistance as I press down on your fist to flex the hand downward toward your inner wrist." As I do this Nick is providing a little force to resist the movement but not enough to prevent the motion.

"Ouch! That hurts." Nick jerks back from the motion of downward wrist flexion as I stretch muscle and tendon structures running from the back of his wrist and hand to his outer or lateral elbow which produces pain at the muscle's insertion point. This test combined with my light pressure at the outer elbow indicates the damage and inflammation associated with his medical diagnosis of 'lateral epicondylitis'.

Medical terms are most often taken from Latin and if we break it down lateral refers to the outer side of the elbow as we are viewed in anatomic position. (In anatomic position the human body is viewed as standing erect, face forward with feet together and hands at our sides with palms facing forward.) The epicondyle refers to two bony knobs at the sides of our elbow. A lateral epicondyle on the outer side and a medial epicondyle on the inner side of the lower portion of our upper arm bone the 'humerus'. 'Itis', added to the end of epicondyle refers to inflammation. So the term lateral epicondylitis is easily understandable and with the advent of the Internet, any medical diagnosis employing 'med-speak' can be referenced and understood by the general public by doing a little research.

"Nick, it's obvious that you have inflammation and damage of the tendons inserting into the elbow. You can never tell for sure if conservative non-surgical therapy will be effective especially since you use your elbow every day making pizza. Is there anyone who can take over for you while we do therapy?"

"Doc, that pizzeria is my baby. How can I take off?"

"If you end up with surgery you'll be out for months."

"Well, I have a cousin who has helped in the past. Let me see what I can do."

"Okay, so no more deep rubbing or stretching of the area. Each time you do that you're making it worse by stretching and disrupting the area and damaging the healing your body is attempting to perform. You're already sleeping properly on your back or left side with a pillow under your arm. I want you to take a six-week break form pizza and if this is not agreeable I won't be able to treat you as you would never heal and even with that you may need more time off. You need to be here six days a week for ultrasound for the next three weeks and at least three times per week after that for three more weeks."

"Why so often?"

"Tendon injuries heal slowly and can easily scar especially if of long duration, which may have already occurred. Ultrasound can soften the scar tissue and heal the area but you will need it daily for a while. Also, you will be using ice packs every hour or two during your waking hours for the next week to two weeks."

"How about my brace?"

"Your brace puts external pressure on the elbow and tendons decreasing the blood flow to the area. We need good blood flow to allow for healing and tissue regeneration so I want you to skip the brace. You can do some very light massage with an ice cube or a frozen cup of water." I instruct Nick to freeze some water in Styrofoam cup, peel away the top half-inch and use the ice in a light massage several times per day for approximately 10 minutes. This will help the area by reducing swelling and stimulating circulation.

Nick Week Three

Nick has now been receiving ultrasound as prescribed, sleeping primarily on his back and doing the ice pack and light ice rub applications. He is feeling better and rates his pain at a 2 on a 10 point pain scale. As the pain has significantly dropped and swelling is lessened it is a good time to being rehabilitative exercise. I direct him to acquire a one pound dumbbell (or other weight) and begin wrist extension exercises. To do these he can simply lay his forearm on a table, grasp the weight and flex the hand backward toward the elbow. These he will continue doing with perhaps 15 repetitions two to three times per day over the next week adding a pound every one to two weeks for four to eight weeks maxing out at three to five pounds. At the end of four to eight weeks, he should be able to resume light duties within the restaurant that do not require stretching the elbow. As there is no sure way to calculate readiness for the resumption of work, common sense and gradual reintegration of workload is recommended over many weeks with careful avoidance of deep stretching activities initially.

Nancy's Aging Spine

Nancy, a lovely woman of 83 years young, hasn't seen a chiropractor in twenty years but now is sitting in my exam room requesting a 'tune-up'. She's been having general spine pain especially in the mid-back for a few months and is quite sure that a couple of adjustments will, "Do the trick", and end her discomfort. My examination indicates otherwise. Lying Nancy face downward on my exam table, I palpate her spine and find the fixation and near-complete rigidity that is often associated with severe osteoarthritis, OA, of the spine. Advanced osteoarthritis of the spine is hallmarked by generalized calcification of the spinal joints and ligaments. In Nancy's case, this is coupled with a severely bowed or kyphotic thoracic spine and forward head position often seen in those with years of side sleeping that can curve the shoulders forward and accelerate the bowing process.

Ordinary forms of spinal manipulation are contraindicated in this situation as the spine is essentially cementing itself in place over time. This certainly is not a good situation and can lead to a host of problems including balance issues and spontaneous fracture or collapse of thoracic vertebrae placed under excessive load by the kyphosis. In the elderly, there is also lessening of bone density due to osteopenia or osteoporosis when the spine has lost mineral content. These all add up to a fragile spine that requires delicate handling. Fortunately, most chiropractors and chiropractic specialists have techniques at their disposal to provide safe and gentle treatment in such cases.

Having Nancy continue lying face downward on my adjusting table I get her permission to employ a series of gentle spine stretches timed with her breathing. As she slowly exhales I apply light pressure to gently stretch her spine from top of the shoulders to the lower back and pelvis. This is repeated several times. At no time is there a forceful thrust or maneuver. Following this, I gently vibrate the spine and spinal joints from upper shoulders to lower back and pelvis running a professional vibrator along the spine for one to two minutes again with a light force of perhaps five pounds. This combination of stretch and vibration is useful to increase spinal flexibility and spinal joint lubrication and may be considered a form of global spinal adjustment. Nancy like most seniors with severe OA has an immediate sense of relief on arising. We will continue in this manner over several sessions as we increase spinal motion and health. If the spine becomes sufficiently flexible with this therapy more aggressive manipulation can be performed. Gentle rehab and back strengthening exercises will be added later and coupled perhaps with light yoga or Tai Chi. I ask Nancy to begin attempting to sleep more on her back which will be difficult for her at first, but will help, even at this late date; to arrest her kyphotic progression.

Sam's 'Cluster' Headaches

Sam, a 42-year-old mechanical engineer spends long hours on engineering projects with his new start-up firm. He has a big job currently that if successfully managed will secure more work to come and set the tone for future business. In the past four months, his twelve-hour days spent doing computer assisted work have been playing hell with his neck and upper back. He takes breaks here and there and tries stretching the neck and asking Alice a long-time friend and co-worker to do a little massage on his neck from time to time. His neck seems to feel better after stretch and massage but within a short time feels tight and painful again. When Alice is too busy to lead him a hand he finds that if he squeezes the upper neck he gets relief for a while. For six weeks now he has been getting right temple pain. It began as some moderate and transient sharp and throbbing pain but has now progressed to a searing pain that may last for hours and encompasses the right eye, face and neck. Now even squeezing his right upper neck at the base of the skull doesn't seem to help but putting ice on the temple or eye eases the pain slightly. The attacks which are daily now are interrupting his concentration and he feels he is falling behind on his engineering deadline.

Not only is he having pain but his right eye is tearing, red and puffy. He is sleeping poorly as well. He often has the onset of severe headache an hour or two after going to bed. He says that sleeping seems to bring on the attacks which may also occur at any point in the day but often onset at about the same time which for Sam is usually 10:30 AM after approximately three hours at his desk.

He has visited his MD and a headache specialist who have examined him and ordered an MRI of the brain which was normal. (Prolonged and severe headaches usually warrant an MRI of the brain but are rarely positive for any underlying abnormality.) Sam has been diagnosed with cluster headaches and placed on oral corticosteroids. Although this medication has reduced the intensity of his pain somewhat, he is concerned about serious side effects such as diabetes, hypertension and cataracts that make them inappropriate for long term use.

The pain of a cluster headache is often described as sharp, penetrating or burning. People with this condition say that the pain feels like a hot poker being stuck in the eye or that the eye is being pushed out of its socket. Some migraine-like symptoms, including nausea, sensitivity to light and sound may occur with a cluster headache, though usually on one side. The exact cause of cluster headaches is unknown. Abnormalities in the hypothalamus have been postulated as a causative factor since unlike other headache forms, cluster headaches may occur at the same approximate time each day which, some suggest, may involve the body's biological clock. In humans, the biological clock is located in the hypothalamus, which lies deep in the center of your brain. Abnormalities of the hypothalamus could explain the timing and cyclical nature of cluster headache. However, as you will soon learn there is a simple and far more logical explanation for these excruciatingly severe and punctual headaches and it involves mechanical stress to the neck.

Unlike migraine and tension headache, cluster headache generally isn't associated with triggers, such as foods, hormonal changes or stress. Once a cluster period begins, however, consumption of alcohol can quickly trigger a splitting headache. For this reason, many people with cluster headaches avoid alcohol as it can be toxic to nerve tissue. Thiamine, folate, niacin, vitamins B6 and B12 and vitamin E are all needed for proper nerve function. Drinking too much can deplete these nutrients and lead to nerve irritation and provoke the start or severity of a headache.

As Sam's story unfolds he constantly rubs his right upper neck, temple and presses into the eye. I know this stimulation helps to block the pain but unfortunately for Sam can be instrumental in his headaches as we will shortly see.

As I begin my examination, I see that Sam has great posture with an erect and well-balanced head situated directly over his shoulder. This, as we have seen, is a good finding because so many people with long hours of computer use, crafting or book work have forward head carriage which as we have seen stresses the neck and may lead to neck, upper back and headache pain.

Asking Sam to sit I palpate his neck. Immediately I note swelling in the rear upper neck on the right side. Probing this area lightly and the skull just above produces severe lancinating pain into the right temple and eye as Sam pulls away from my probing finger.

"That's hurts like hell!"

"Sorry Sam. I'm just trying to figure this out." As I palpate I also detect that Sam has a major shift in the uppermost cervical vertebrae, known as the atlas. The atlas is an important vertebra as it basically holds the head in two saucer or cup-like joint surfaces that accept the bony knobs or 'condyles' at the rearward base of the skull. The atlas and the vertebra just below it 'the axis' account for half of the flexion, extension and rotation of our neck and head. Imaging a thin ring-like bone four centimeters front to back and six centimeters long able to support a twelve-pound head while allowing the head and neck to rotate, flex and extend! This while allowing the brain stem and spinal cord to pass through its inner ring.

Unfortunately, the atlas misalignment I'm detecting in Sam's case is a leading cause of headache as it produces stress to the soft tissue of the upper neck including the brain stem and the major occipital nerves exiting the upper spine and running just below the scalp to the temple and eye region. Atlas misalignment or 'subluxation' is common after seemingly minor sports or other injuries. It also occurs in infants who experience a strenuous delivery. It's common in stomach sleepers and those who spend long hours in head flexion at work, school or play. The fact that light pressure at the base of the skull so dramatically provokes Sam's pain is a prime indicator that disturbance here may be the culprit in Sam's cluster headache diagnosis and strongly suggests he has been misdiagnosed and is suffering from occipital nerve pain also known as 'occipital neuralgia' instead of cluster headaches.

An occipital nerve block can be useful for temporary relief of occipital neuralgia until proper therapy and spinal correction reduces swelling and improves vertebral position with chiropractic spinal manipulation. This is performed by injecting a numbing agent (anesthetic) and corticosteroid into the area around the emergence of the occipital nerve, located at the back of your head.

To better understand the problem a little anatomy lesson is needed. Cervical vertebrae are often numbered for convenience. The atlas or uppermost vertebrae is C1. The axis just below is C2 and so on. The greater and lesser occipital nerves originate on both the right and left side of the upper neck between the 1st, 2nd and 3rd or uppermost cervical vertebrae .

Occipital neuralgia occurs due to irritation or trauma of the occipital nerves (ON). It can be caused by an auto accident where the head impacts the headrest or other injuries of the upper neck or scalp. Other causes may include degenerative changes of the upper cervical spine at C1-C2 or C2- C3.

In this case, Sam is his own worst enemy. "Sam you have occipital neuralgia. From your history, it would seem that your neck became tight with work and your habit of rubbing your upper neck, where the occipital nerves emerge, has exacerbated the problem. This habit has progressively bruised and irritated the occipital nerves over time. The more you massaged the area the worse the pain became and so the more you massaged to relieve it."

"You're saying I did this to myself?"

"Yes."

"So where do we go from here."

"We are going to do therapy to reduce the swelling and irritation of the general area and the nerve tissue. We also have to do some cervical spine manipulation to re-center your atlas which has shifted to the right."

"My what?"

"Sam, not only are the tissues and nerves swollen in your upper neck and scalp, you have a misalignment of the uppermost vertebra in the neck. It's known as the atlas and in your case has shifted to the right. This malposition further irritates the nerves and the many muscles they pass through as they weave their way up to the scalp. Combining therapy such as ultrasound and ice packs to reduce swelling in this area along with spinal manipulation of the atlas to reposition this vertebra in its normal position will help to alleviate the soft tissue and nerve irritation producing your pain."

"Is spinal manipulation painful?"

"Sometimes a little when you're so tender in the upper neck but nothing compared to the pain you have been experiencing."

"Is it safe?"

"Extremely safe. My malpractice costs are a small fraction of what your primary doctor pays."

Following ultrasound and cold packs, I have Sam lie face up on the table. "Sam, I'd like to adjust (manipulate) your atlas to start the process of better centering the vertebra. Since your atlas has shifted to the right I'm going to apply a moderate force to the right side of the vertebra to move it leftward and toward its normal position. Centering the vertebra will diminish pressure on the occipital nerves. Over time as we continue the adjustments we should be able to completely reposition the atlas. The movement I apply with my hands, (some doctors use instrumentation), will be quick and because the spinal vertebrae have joints, will create a sound similar to the pop when you pull a finger to stretch a joint. Is that acceptable?"

"Are you sure it's safe?"

"Sam, I've done these adjustments thousands of times and never had a problem.

Getting Sam's approval I place my right hand in contact with his misaligned atlas and applying a quick and very precise force move the vertebrae toward its central/normal position. Sam feels the movement which is completed in about a tenth of a second.

As I help Sam sit up he's smiling. "That's it?"

"Just a little fine-tuning."

"Wow, that wasn't painful!"

"Most often it's not."

Although occipital neuralgia can be extremely debilitating its resolution, in my experience, is easily accomplished with correct therapy, including correcting forward head posture in some individuals. Proper ergonomics and postural changes are also needed at home and in the workplace. Patient interaction has convinced me that occipital neuralgia is quite common and often misdiagnosed as cluster headache. Although the normal course of treatment may span a few weeks I have little doubt that Sam will do well with conservative care.

Mary's Knee Pain and Bunions

Mary, a full-time bartender for the past eight years and now in her thirties, has increasingly severe right knee pain. She had an MRI two months ago and a small medial (inner knee) meniscal tear was noted in the cartilage. Her orthopedist recommended strengthening exercises with a PT for six weeks at three times per week. She attended the PT which helped but now two weeks later the pain has returned with pain in her hip and outer thigh. As she gives me the history she sits with her right foot resting on its outer edge and splays the right knee out at an odd angle while rubbing her right thigh.

Pain patients universally stretch and rub painful areas as these maneuvers interrupt the sensation of pain messages to the brain and temporarily warm and loosen the painful area to the detriment of the underlying injury itself. I ask Mary to straighten the right leg and foot, placing her foot flatly on the floor and to stop the rubbing as I explain why.

"Mary, in what positions do you sleep and what do you do to try to lessen your pain."

"Well, I sleep on my sides and when the pain is bad I stretch and take ibuprofen."

"Does that help?"

"The ibuprofen helps for a few hours but it's starting to hurt my stomach. Stretching loosens up the area for a while but it seems to be getting worse. At first, it was just the knee pain but now my thigh is hurting and I can feel my low back on the right side getting sore as well."

"Do you limp or favor your gait when you walk?"

"Yeah, it's hard not to."

"Your orthopedist didn't want to do surgery? Did he ask you about sleep positions?"

"No he never ask me how I slept and he said the tear was small and he preferred to wait for now."

Asking Mary to partially disrobe and to put on a gown while I step out, I return to begin the exam. As Mary stands I see that she has pronounced flat feet and stands with her ankles 'pronated' or rolling inward. She also has large bunions at the base of each large toe. As a result of the pronation, she exhibits an inward deviation of both knees in a somewhat knock-kneed posture. Bending to touch her right knee I note that the knee is painful to touch on the inside and somewhat puffy or swollen here. The right lateral leg is also swollen from the outer knee all the way up to the hip. Deeper finger pressure produces pain and avoidance.

"How long have you had the bunions?"

"Since I was a teen."

I have Mary stand in front of a full-length mirror I have in my exam room and point out her inward ankle pronation and inward knee deviation.

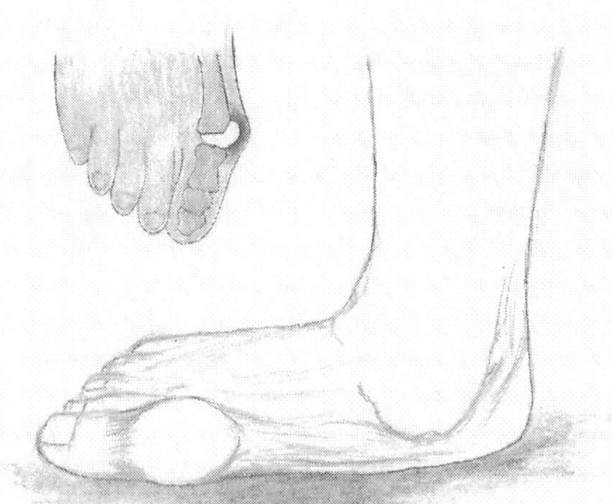

Flat feet and ankle inturning leads to bunion development and wears all the joints of the hips and lower extremities.

"Mary you have a fairly common problem. When you pronate as severely as you do, you create a stress on the foot known as a 'ground reaction' which moves the large toe inward, irritating the large joint at the base of the toe. This stress creates pain and inflammation of the joint and will eventually lead to the formation of bunions. This position also stresses the knee. Pronation forces the knee to deviate inward as you stand or walk. When you first step onto your heal your foot is basically in neutral but as you shift your full weight onto the foot in mid-stance your foot rolls inward and so does the knee. This circular motion is damaging to the cartilage of the knee and may have been responsible for the tear.

A secondary stress is created when you limp. You try to quickly get off the painful leg when walking but what you're really doing is jarring the knee, leg and back as you come down hard and fast on the painful leg. You have to begin to walk smoothly, transitioning your weight gently and without limping if you expect the knee and leg to heal. We're going to begin ultrasound therapy and ice packs on the knee and thigh but more importantly, you will need prescription shoe orthotics to correct the foot pronation and de-stress the knees."

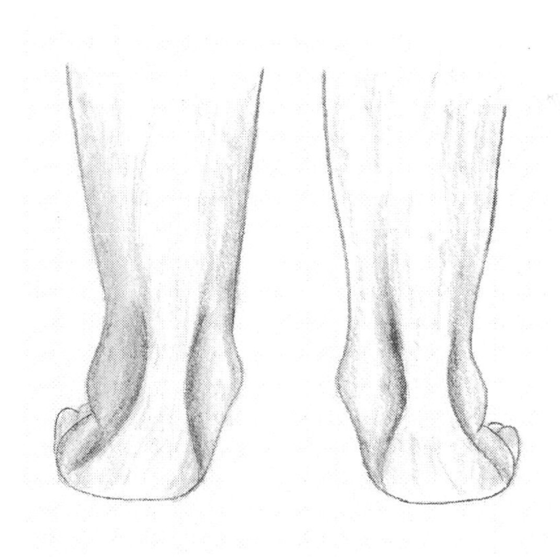

Foot and ankle pronation

Pronation's Pandora's Box

Marked ankle pronation usually coupled with loss of the

foot's normal arch (flat feet) is a leading cause of instability and pain. Pronation has also been implicated in anterior cruciate and posterior cruciate (ACL/PCL) ligament and meniscal (cartilage) tears of the knee. Pronation will ultimately lead to the formation of bunions, fasciitis of the foot, metatarsalgia (pain at the base of the inner toes), ankle strain, shin splints, Achilles tendonitis, radicular nerve pain of the foot and arthritic changes of the hip, knee and foot joints. Pronation results in an altered gait that will stress and damage the low back as well. Pronation should be taken seriously and corrected with exercises and shoe orthotics in all cases.

Shoe Orthotics....Proper Support for the Foot, Knee, Hip and Back

Custom shoe orthotics can be formulated by the orthopedist, podiatrist or chiropractor and are needed when severe pronation or other foot abnormalities exist. However, in minor cases where a prescription orthotic is not indicated, a good 'off the shelf' shoe insert can be purchased at most shoe outlets. If this is the case look for the best 'highest' arch you can find and make sure to remove the insole that came with your shoe so as not to add extra bulk to the insole area when using the new orthotic insert.

Postural Considerations for Knee Complaints

Rule number one is don't stretch the knee and this means postures of sleep and sitting are important. If you're sleeping on the side always have a pillow between the knees and if sleeping with the injured knee uppermost make sure the knee stays on the pillow. If you're lying on your back have one pillow under the knees. Sit straight with knees uncrossed and knees and feet in front of you, bent 90 degrees and on the floor. No twisting the knee and no propping the feet on a stool or hassock with the knee joint unsupported and 'hanging in space'. Also avoid excessive and strenuous exercises which might include running, hiking or biking until proper treatment has reduced your pain scale number to a 1 or 2 on the analog scale and you have made the corrective changes to stabilize the knee discussed above.

Visit HealingTheHumanMachine.com for a video demonstrating strengthening exercises for the knee and leg.

Any significant joint pathology might require surgical intervention but one should always try to treat conservatively if possible, for at least six weeks observing all the appropriate dos and don'ts that are mentioned in this book. With proper adherence to these principals, surgery may be avoided.

Further Considerations for Knee Pain

The knee is distinct from the other major load-bearing joints in that soft tissues rather than the 'fit' of the joining bones primarily stabilize the knee. Here the upper femur or thigh bone meets the lower tibial bone, the connecting contours of each being somewhat dissimilar, they require large horseshoe-shaped pads, the lateral and medial meniscus, interposed between to help them match up. Another important difference is the patella, a small oval bone connected to the massive muscles of the upper thigh required to slide through the femoral groove, a depression on the front of the femur requiring normal alignment of the knee to track properly. The knee is stabilized by two broad lateral and medial 'collateral' ligaments spanning the joint and two internal ligaments the anterior and posterior 'cruciate' all required to control stability and prevent slippage of this highly complex structure.

Added to this innate instability, walking or jogging increases the forces on the knee significantly, increasing as much as 2 to 3 times our body weight (BW)! Golf may increase this to 4xBW on the leading foot and squatting with weights can increase the force to 5-6xBW! Obesity takes its toll on all our joints but especially the knee; five pounds of excess weight becomes fifteen pounds on the knee in motion! Now consider that in many activities we 'plant' the foot to execute upper body movements increasing vectors of force via angulation and rotation of the knee. It's a pure wonder that this magnificent joint holds up as well as it does!

Biomechanical faults are commonly seen in those with knee pain. Inward deviation of the knee known as a 'valgus' deformity may be mild or pronounced and is a common finding often associated with ankle pronation. By contrast, an outward deviation of the knee known as a 'varus' deformity is less common. Either will usually result in abnormal knee wear.

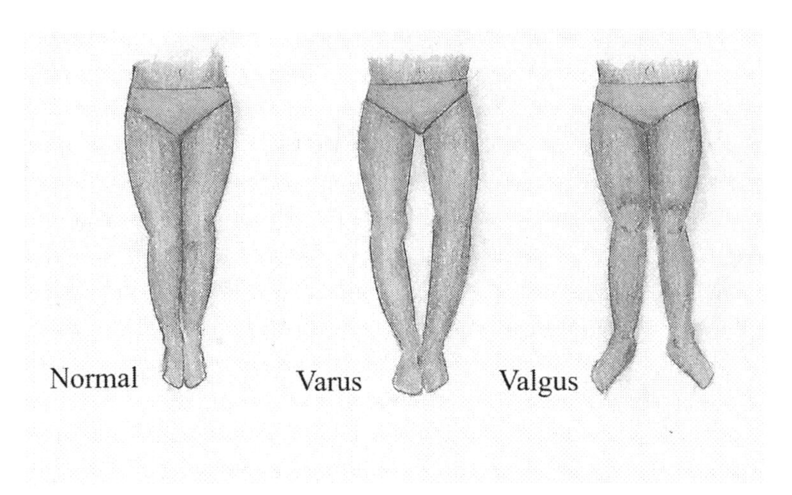

The most common cause of knee pain results from knee strain; usually in the form of a mild to moderate medial collateral ligament tear. Here we find that the inner 'strap' ligament of the knee spanning the joint and attaching the upper leg bone or 'femur' to the lower leg bone the 'tibia', has been damaged by diffuse filament tearing. This is an incomplete tear and usually heals well if managed properly. Knee valgus is often associated with this injury (and most other complaints of the knee).

Knee requires proper support and stabilization and in a moment we'll discuss the Victory Knee Brace. Arthritis, cruciate tears and tears of the lateral and medial meniscus can frequently occur as well. Again, using some common sense is the best way to proceed. If a painful knee is usable with a fair to good range of motion and reasonable strength then waiting four to six weeks while using the strategies for knee posture and conservative therapy discussed in this book should reduce pain and improve function. Following this regimen and then beginning home rehab with strengthening exercises, begun when the pain has diminished, will continue improvement typically. Of course, evaluating underlying causes of knee stress like ankle/foot pronation, internal femoral rotation and leg length difference should be given major consideration if present and approached/corrected accordingly.

If knee pain is more severe and there is a significant limitation of motion or function then diagnostic tests such as x-ray and possibly MRI are in order. Arthritis will vary by degree and mild to moderate arthritis of the knee often responds to rest, the non-compressive and non-stretching postures I endorse along with ultrasound therapy. Taking curcumin, discussed later on, can be extremely helpful. In cases of arthritis, a heating pad may be substituted for ice, (however, ice packs often work just as well). In severe cases of arthritis demonstrated on x-ray or MRI, surgical intervention may be indicated and this should be discussed with a competent orthopedic surgeon. If imaging should disclose a cruciate ligament tear or significant (large) meniscal tear, surgery is usually indicated.

The knee is somewhat unique as it is prone to arthritic change both in the knee joint proper and in the area under the knee cap or 'patellae'. Arthritic change under the knee cap begins as simple inflammation and progresses to 'chondromalacia patellae', a softening of the cartilage beneath the knee cap that will lead through several stages to the degenerative changes and calcified debris associated with this condition. Chondromalacia is nearly always caused by irregular movement patterns of the kneecap usually related to an inward deviation of the knee and often foot/ankle pronation. Chondromalacia may also be related to abnormal hip alignment. Both should be evaluated by a professional. As we have learned, long term mechanical issues have a profound wearing effect on the body and how well it holds up.

Visit HealingTheHumanMachine.com for a video discussing these topics.

The Victory Knee Brace

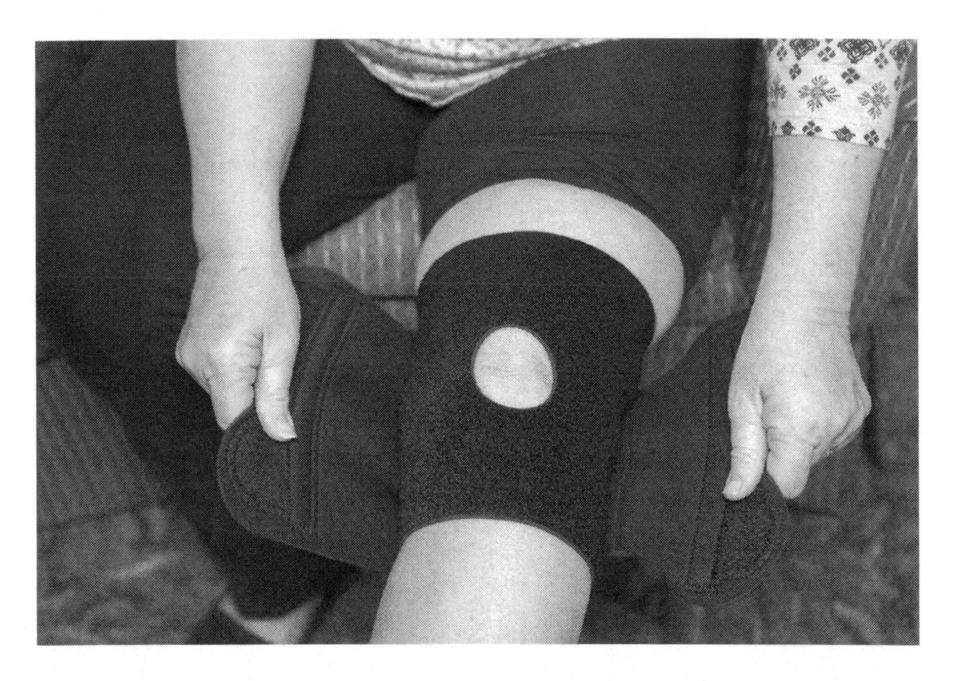

I invented the Victory Knee Brace for its easy ability to position and secure. Once slipped over the foot and leg the two side tabs can be quickly opened, brace positioned and fastened by extending and securing the two side tabs simultaneously due to its unique interwoven design. The Victory Brace allows for free movement of the knee while providing excellent compression to limit swelling and instability. It is quite comfortable and the neoprene fabric provides major warmth and support for the knee. My patients tell me it is the most comfortable knee brace they have ever worn.

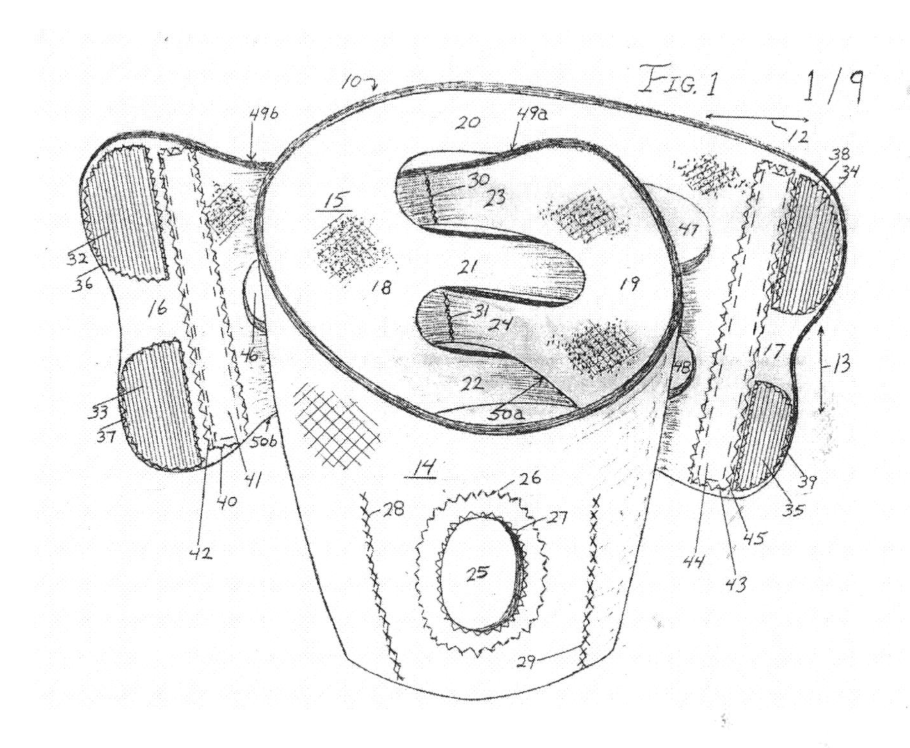

Visit HealingTheHumanMachine.com for a video demonstrating the Victory Knee Brace or to order one.

Gail's 'Fibromyalgia' and Scoliosis

Gail moves somewhat haltingly with obvious pain in or about the low back and seats herself gingerly in my exam room to begin her story of diffuse and chronic pain diagnosed as fibromyalgia. Now at 36 years of age, Gail began experiencing knee and back pain as a twelve-year-old and was at that time diagnosed with scoliosis having a 12-degree 'levo' or left, lumbar and thoracic scoliotic curve. In her late teens, she began to have pain in the neck and upper back which occasionally traveled into her upper arms. Now she has constant arm pain and posterior skull and headache pain. She has seen her M.D., two orthopedists, gone for PT and one chiropractor all with little relief.

Fibromyalgia (FM) is a medical condition characterized by chronic widespread pain and a heightened and painful response to pressure at multiple 'pressure points'. Symptoms other than pain may occur, leading to the use of the term fibromyalgia syndrome (FMS). These may include feeling tired to a degree that normal activities are affected, as well as sleep disturbance and joint stiffness. Some people also report difficulty with swallowing, bowel and bladder abnormalities, numbness and tingling of extremities and poor cognitive performance. Fibromyalgia is frequently associated with depression, anxiety and stress-related disorders such as post-traumatic stress disorder, PTSD. Not all people with fibromyalgia experience all the associated symptoms and may instead have a 'mixed bag' of these complaints.

Medical texts will tell you that fibromyalgia's exact cause is unknown but is believed to involve psychological, genetic, neurobiological and environmental factors. It is interesting to note that the same areas of fibromyalgia pain are the very same common areas for musculoskeletal pain. Could it be that fibromyalgia is simply a body experiencing a collection of biomechanical defects and postural stresses that have been affecting the body for so long that pain becomes ingrained in the body and facilitated by the mind?

"Gail, so why are you picking on me?

"I'm sorry?"

"Well, you've seen everyone else why me?"

"My girlfriend said you were good."

"You know, you can't believe everything you hear." I smile as she laughs at that and we begin to establish a little rapport.

"Do you have any x-rays taken of your back, neck or knees?"

Fortunately, she has come with radiology reports and three discs containing x-ray images of the neck and back as well as an MRI of the knee. The radiology reports from three years ago indicate mild straightening of the cervical spine, thoracic scoliosis and some 'effusion' (or swelling), of the knees without other pathology. As I look at the studies I agree with most of the findings but the neck is not mildly straight but slightly reversed. Unfortunately, the lumbar spine x-ray study is 'collimated' and only the immediate spine and the very top of the pelvis can be seen. Typically, collimated x-rays visualize only the spinal vertebrae of the scoliotic curves themselves and perhaps a small portion of the pelvis and ribs. The entire pelvis, hips and upper legs remain unseen. Since the majority of scoliosis cases I've encountered are due to leg length differences or abnormalities of hip or pelvic formation and balance, such information is needed. I can see that the sacrum appears low on the left side but I am unable to explain why this should be without a full non-collimated x-ray.

"Gail, the studies don't look so bad but we will need another AP lumbar x-ray to see your upper legs to access leg length equality." I ask Gail to explain her habits and how she tries to manage her pain. As she does I note the many soft tissue healing rules she breaks each day; stomach and side sleeping, resting her feet on a stool with her knees hanging in space, sitting on the floor Indian style, limping in pain, lots of stretch, lots of computer work and lots of massage to any painful spot.

"Okay, let's do an exam." I hand her a gown and explain the need to visualize both her limbs and torso asking her to remove her outer garments while I leave the room. (I usually suggest that my female patients may have a female staff member present while we do the exam. Very few require it.)

When I re-enter, I ask Gail to stand with her back to me and feet roughly twelve inches apart and on the same parallel line as I part the gown to inspect her posture. Both knees deviate inward slightly as do both feet with collapse of the foot arches producing pronation. What's most striking is that Gail's left pelvic area seems lower than the right. There is a definite tilt or downward inclination of the pelvis from right to left and her spine does appear to curve toward the downward side. When viewing Gail's posture from the side the shoulders are bowed and carried forward as is her head. She definitely has compromised posture and I let her know.

As I palpate the neck, shoulders, lower back, buttock and knee areas with lightly probing fingers there are multiple tender areas. I explain my findings and tell Gail we're going to begin ultrasound and ice packs to the neck and lower back. I'm holding off on any spinal manipulation until I see the non-collimated weight bearing (standing) x-rays of the lumbar/pelvis and upper femur heads (tops of her legs as they meet the hip). "Gail when you get your x-rays you'll be standing with your feet 10-12 inches apart. While I would like to have the full x-ray films for examination and measurement, if the facility is unable to give you films a CD will do." I give her a lot of do's and don'ts for home care and posture and re-schedule her next treatment for two days later to allow her time to get the x-ray as I hand her a prescription.

Gail Day Two

Gail re-enters with the erect lumbar spine x-ray. The study I'm reviewing was done on a 14x17 inch x-ray film that allows us to see her lumbar spine, pelvis and her upper femurs (leg bones). Placing the x-ray on a lighted view box I take a few moments to do some careful measurements.

"Gail, your left leg is approximately 13mm or 1/2 inch shorter than your right leg. I'm sure you can easily understand that your spine and 24 movable spinal bones are constantly balanced atop the pelvis. Abnormalities of pelvic or leg length development can create an unlevel base for the spine. The flexible spine will naturally curve toward the lower side as the upper torso shifts it's weight to the opposite longer leg side to attain balance. This is a completely natural reaction to imbalance and simply a 'functional adaptation' of the spine to resting on an unlevel base. The good news in your case is that your spinal curve has not progressed in the last three years and if you're willing we can formulate orthotics for both feet but lift or elevate the left orthotic on the short leg side to help level the pelvis and reduce your spinal curve. This will reduce stress on the spine helping to prevent degenerative changes to the spinal discs, spinal joints and hips; joints that are being mechanically stressed by your leg length disparity. This should also alleviate some of your pain."

"Could I only use one for the left shoe or just a heel lift?"

"No. You'll have a lifted left and non-lifted right orthotic. It's important to have both as we want your gait to be smooth, even and symmetrical. The value of a podiatric grade orthotic is that unlike a heel lift alone the orthotic incorporates the lift but also supports the arch and foot properly. A heel lift alone doesn't support the arch and basically leaves your mid-foot unsupported and stressed as we stand or walk. We don't want to cause you more problems."

Gail Week Six

"Gail, how do you feel?"

"Well compared to how I did feel, I feel great!"

Gail has now been wearing the lifted left and non-lifted right orthotic for three weeks and sleeping on her back. She stopped stretching and uses a pillow under her knees when in bed. We've been using ultrasound in therapy and gentle spinal adjustments to increase spinal mobility and improve spinal alignment. She is still occasionally using the ice packs but less and less so. Her pain scale number has diminished to a 1-2 and all complaints have lessened.

I will now start her on the neck exercises with the 'Neck Correct'. In the examination, I can see that her left hip and pelvis seem much more level with her shoe orthotics in place and the scoliotic curve seems less severe as well. As she is feeling so much better we will avoid having more x-rays done at this point to evaluate the lumbar spine as there is a small risk of excessive x-ray and I am satisfied that the orthotics are doing their job. I'll get another cervical lateral or side view x-ray in approximately six months to check for cervical curve improvement with the Neck Correct exercises.

"Okay kiddo, we have another problem to tackle."

Gail's Growing 'Dowager's Hump'

"Gail I'm sure you've seen elderly men or women that are bent over when erect and can't straighten; it's as if their spine is permanently curved and fused in a bowed manner."

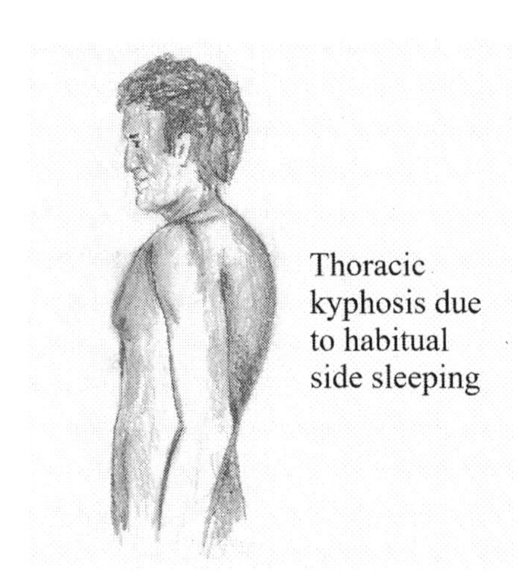

Gail's eyes widen a little; "You're talking about my grandmother. At first, it was just a little but now she can't straighten at all. I feel so sorry for her. When I talk to her she can barely look up! My mother has a little of the same problem but not nearly as bad."

"That's what I'm talking about, a condition called a 'Dowager's Hump. Do you know how your mother and grandmother sleep?"

"I'm really not sure."

"Want to make a bet? I'm going to write the position they sleep in on a piece of paper, seal it in an envelope and place it in your file.

On your next visit, we'll open the envelope together. If I'm right about both you buy me a bagel and a cup of coffee if not I'll treat you. Deal?"

"Deal!"

Gail enters three days later with a grin and tells me she has been checking on both her mother and grandmother each night and both are side sleepers.

"Okay, open the envelope."

Looking at the paper Gail is surprised, "How did you know?"

"Because I have asked every woman or man who has entered my practice for the past twenty-five years what position they sleep in when they have bowed shoulders, a precursor to 'Dowager's Hump', and everyone has been a side sleeper. Want to hear an interesting story? Many years ago I treated a German couple with the most beautiful erect posture. One day we were discussing mattresses and the older gentleman said that in Germany the mattresses were thin and most people including his wife and he slept on these mattresses placed directly on the floor and on their backs! I have taken note of every stooped shouldered patient since then. Gail, while it's too late for your grandmother it may not be too late for your mom and it's certainly not too late for you!" I let the statement hang and I see the light of recognition in Gail's eyes.

"Oh my God! I'm a side sleeper!"

"Yes and the weight of your torso is slowly shaping and shifting your shoulders forward. As that happens, more and more downward force is acting on your mid-back and thoracic spine to increase its curvature. As this condition accelerates soon your neck and head are moving forward as well further increasing the curve force on the thoracic spine. It's like a snowball rolling downhill, getting bigger and picking up speed."

"What can I do?"

"What the German couple did; sleep on your back on a firm mattress and stay off your side. I'll also give you exercises to strengthen and stretch your back and chest area while the Neck Correct exercises will help to move your head into a more erect position."

"I always thought having a back curve was about too little

calcium or vitamin D and something to do with osteoporosis."

"They certainly play a part since a lack of vitamin D and poor mineral intake can weaken bone. This makes the spinal bones more porous increasing the likelihood of osteoporosis weakening them. This can lead to a compression fracture of the thoracic spine as the compressional forces increase with spinal bowing and poor posture.

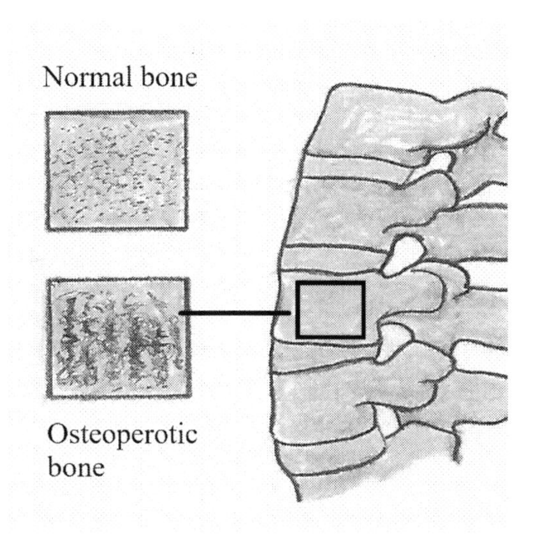

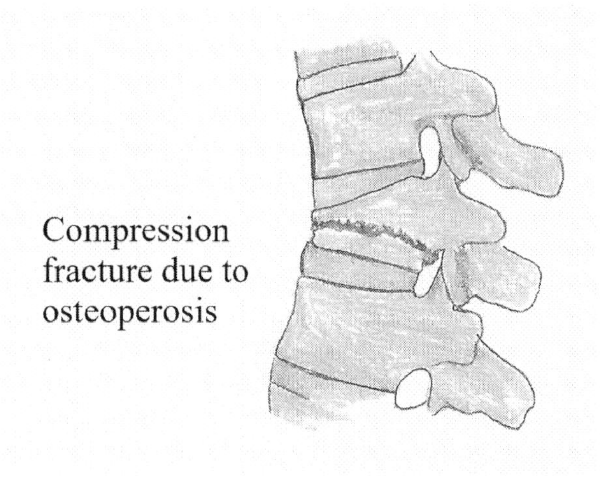

Chronic side sleeping with the weight of your torso on

the downward shoulder structures slowly shapes and bows your shoulders forward. Simultaneously the head and neck move forward as well, creating a bowed and slumped posture. As that happens slowly over time, an ever-increasing downward force is acting on your mid-back and thoracic spine to accelerate curvature. The aging spine often weakened by osteoporotic bone loss and increasingly stressed and overloaded by the added forces of bad posture is at risk for spontaneous fracture and collapse of thoracic vertebrae. Thus begins the process of 'Dowager's Hump' formation. Each successive and painful compression fracture accelerating the condition.

Spinal and Biomechanical Conditions

A Common Reason for Chronic Low Back Pain: 'Lumbar Compression Syndrome' of Facet Joints and Spinous Processes

The low back can be understood more easily if we simplify the lumbar spine down to just five vertebrae, with multiple joints and the interposed discs separating them. Of course, there are lots of small and large muscles attached to the vertebrae by tendons as well but to keep it simple let's acknowledge that these can be damaged or torn with trauma and ignore them for now and look at a different source of low back pain.

The discs separating the vertebrae are composed of a strong and resilient matrix of outer retaining fibers known as the 'annulus' and an inner 'nucleus'. The nucleus is a round fluid-filled 'ball-bearing' shape in the center acting as a pivot point for the vertebrae which is contained by the tough outer annulus. The disc has a high fluid content normally but with age or with injury the disc can lose fluid, thin and wear. A thick healthy disc allows for good separation of the vertebrae and the delicate spinal joints (facets) between the vertebrae. With disc thinning however these joints, similar to those of the fingers, can become overloaded, swollen and painful.

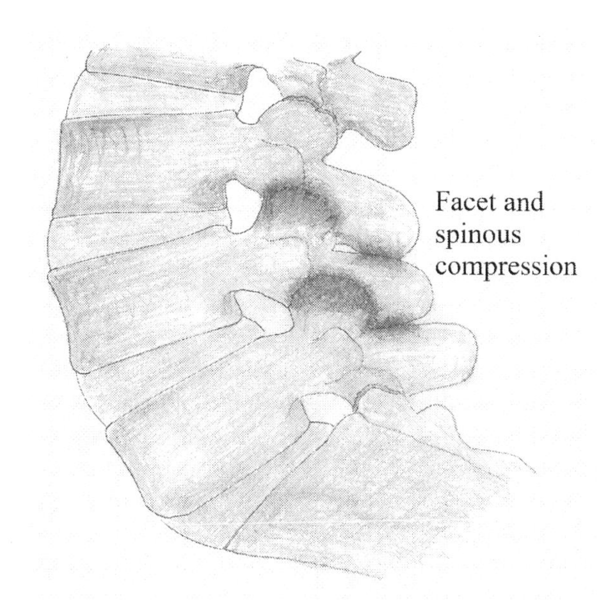

Vertebrae also have bony projections for the attachment of muscles and tendons. One such projection is the spinous process, a vertical, fin-like bone coming straight off the back of each vertebra. Normally there is a little space between each spinous but some people have large spinous projections that touch or jam into each other, especially with disc narrowing. Compounding this problem is obesity. The more belly weight we carry the more our low backs jam due to the tendency of excess tummy fat to increase lumbar curvature or lordosis. (Wearing high heel shoes does the same.)

Lordosis is the natural and normal forward curvature that all low backs should have but excessive lordosis can be a problem in people of all ages even with healthy discs. Excessive lordosis brings the rearward components of the lumbar spine in closer contact increasing facet and spinous compression. Abnormalities of spinal balance can also add to compressive phenomena as unleveling often promotes jamming of spinal structures on the concave side of lateral spinal curves often associated with scoliosis. So, in fact, multiple factors can lead to spinous and joint compression making it by far the most common structural reason for low back pain that I and many colleagues term 'Lumbar Compression Syndrome'.

Identifying spinous and facet joint compression as a source of your back pain is fairly easy; if when standing for just a few minutes you begin to develop low-grade central spine pain, pressure, or a burning sensation that begins to radiate into one but usually both upper buttocks, you likely have this problem. Many people with this condition constantly shift their weight from leg to leg. Weight-bearing low back x-rays easily reveal this condition.

The good news is that lumbar compression and lordosis can be lessened with specific exercises to target weakened muscles and tight pelvic structures. This isn't a quick fix but if you do the exercises daily within four to six weeks there should be a reduction in pain as the strengthened muscles begin to reduce lordosis. After three months of daily exercise, you should be able to reduce the frequency of exercise to three times per week. During the first few weeks wearing a snug to tight lumbar support belt will lessen pain while support muscles are becoming stronger.

Visit HealingTheHumanMachine.com for a video of my preferred exercises to tame lumbar lordosis.

The interesting thing about lumbar compression of facet joints and spinous processes is that you only have to reduce lordosis slightly to significantly reduce the pain of over- compression of these structures. Staying lean and keeping up with the exercises are key.

Disc Protrusions and Herniations

As we discussed the disc separating each spinal vertebra is a strong and resilient matrix of outer retaining fibers known as the annulus and an inner core or nucleus. With age or trauma, the annulus can begin to form minute cracks that may evoke no or only minor back pain. These changes are the result of simple aging, chronic bad posture, minor injuries or excessive forces in lifting or sports. These cracks may weaken the disc producing a diffuse bulging or protrusion of the disc, which if sufficiently large, can contact and pressurize the spinal cord or nerves. Should disc tearing be more severe, the nucleus can be partially displaced causing a more distinct nodular type 'herniation' which can again trap and pressurize a spinal nerve, the spinal cord or both. Thus the tale of the man who bends over to pick up a pencil or sneezes and succumbs to a disc herniation represents that one extra force that overloaded a weakened disc. Of course, even in a younger spine, excessive loading may result in disc herniation.

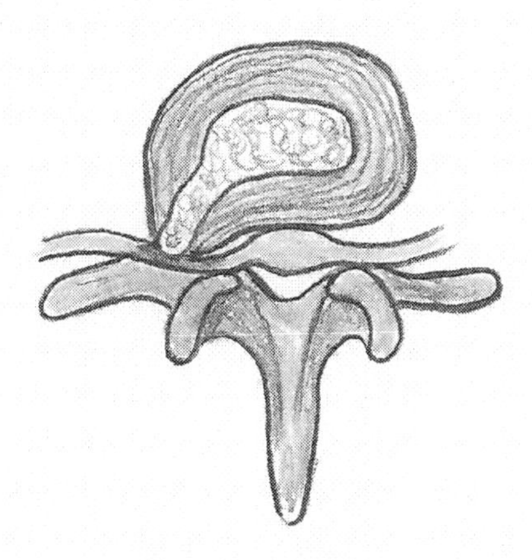

Lumbar disc herniation with nerve compression

Disc protrusions and herniations can be quite benign as long as they don't significantly compress delicate neural tissue, ie: a spinal nerve or the spinal cord itself. When they do however any number of nasty symptoms may result! Nerves pressured by disc herniations in the cervical spine chiefly affect the arms and those of the low back the legs, sexual organs, bladder or bowels. Symptoms may include lost or diminished deep tendon reflexes, severe linear pain into the arm/hand or leg/foot with numbness, weakness, loss of function and even blood flow changes. Often nerve and cord compressions can be felt as hot, shocking or burning sensations. Lumbar disc herniations can lead to loss of libido, faulty erection and orgasm in men, diminished libido and orgasm in women, difficult and painful urination or defecation, bladder leakage and even infertility.

However, the disc annulus may tear multiple times over many

years and never truly herniate. Any acute lumbar disc injury is often associated with severe low back pain and often an involuntary and uncontrollable tilting or listing of the torso forward or to one side, a condition known as 'antalgia'. This may signal either a full-blown herniation or simply a significant annular tear without true herniation. In instances of an annular tear with or without herniation, severe pain will usually prompt the afflicted to seek out my help but with proper therapy and rest the majority of these patients are typically better within a couple of weeks.

The major indicator of the severity of disc injury from a purely clinical standpoint, (not using MRI scanning), is the severity of symptoms. Severe spinal pain with radicular pain or organ dysfunction calls for an MRI to assess disc status or other pathology. If your MRI indicates no or only a minor degree of disc pathology with little or no spinal cord or nerve compression conservative therapy should be continued. If the MRI indicates major disc pathology then treatment choice is again one of severity.

Good research indicates that lumbar spine traction, usually done in a reciprocal fashion of stretch and unloading of the spine, can be extremely effective in reducing disc herniations without surgery. In a study by Dr. Thomas Gionis and fellow researchers, they state, "Results showed 86% of 219 patients who completed traction therapy reported immediate resolution of symptoms, while 84% remained pain-free 90 days post-treatment. Physical examination findings showed improvement in 92% of the 219 patients and remained intact in 89% of these patients 90 days after treatment."[84] These results have been duplicated many times.[85,86]

In closing, I have used traction in the treatment of hundreds of herniated disc cases and I have recommended many patients to surgery as well. The risk of worsening disc symptoms through traction is minimal but can't be totally discounted. The risk of problems arising from disc surgery is very real including infection, nerve damage, paralysis or even death. Keep in mind however that the choice of treatment is your choice, which should only be made with all the diagnostic facts at hand. A trained and competent physician be it medical or chiropractic should be your guide as you weigh your options understanding that inordinate delay in reducing a large disc herniation can lead to permanent nerve or organ damage.

Also remember, that just because a disc herniation is seen on MRI it may have been present for some time and not the cause of your acute or chronic pain as was discussed in the section 'Overtreating Back Pain...A Profitable Business'.

Disc Degeneration and Spinal Instability

The spine is encased in ligaments. These ligaments span and surround the entire spine attaching to the margins of the spinal vertebra. The healthy, thick and fluid-filled disc, acts as a spacer to hold the vertebrae apart, unloading spinal joints and keeping the encompassing spinal ligaments taunt much like a circus tent pole holds the canvas erect and tight as the guy wires and ropes (ligaments) stabilize the structure.[87] The healthy disc also allows for smooth and stable spinal movement. Disc degeneration changes this equation. A lifetime of load and use on our spinal shock-absorbing discs results in slowly progressing disc fatigue, fluid loss and eventual thinning of these important structures. Major trauma with disc herniation or protrusion will lead to similar changes, only faster. The dehydrated discs, thinner than normal, can no longer keep the ligaments taunt and spinal joints apart. Bending, twisting, coughing, lifting and any of a hundred different actions can result in slippage of spinal vertebrae resulting in pain and compression of delicate spinal structures including spinal nerves. Compressed or 'pinched' spinal nerves like the spark plug wires to our car or the electrical wiring to our house, when disrupted, will begin to alter the function of their target organs! As we have discussed this shifting is termed 'subluxation' by chiropractors. Subluxated vertebrae may be fixed or locked in position or conversely be subject to abnormal movement patterns.

Disc thinning overloads the spinal joints which are normally separated by the thick healthy disc. In the healthy spine, our spinal joints are usually unloaded but due to combined compression changes related to movement may assume 12 to 16% of our body load. However, with disc degeneration the lumbar joint load may increase to 70%![88] Daily over-compression of the spinal joints will lead to the destruction of the delicate membranes of the joint or 'synovium' which produce lubricating joint fluid. With continued joint pressure and destruction the joint will experience arthritic changes as the joint dries up and calcified deposits begin to form. Eventually, severe osteoarthritis can develop with bony spurs around the joint margins known as 'osteophytes'. Progression of these changes can lead to loss of spinal motion and pain. The process is hallmarked by progressive spinal pain and the sensation of 'grit' or of a grinding sensation of spinal joints in movement. This is especially noticeable in the neck or 'cervical spine'.

When vertebrae become locked in abnormal positions or movement patterns due to subluxation or arthritic changes, chiropractic manipulation can improve vertebral placement and functional movement. Adhesions and scar tissue often associated with spinal degeneration can be gently stretched with spinal manipulation affording a lessening of pressures on delicate nerve fibers and increased blood flow to innervate nerve tissue. This reduction in nerve compression can have a restorative effect on organ function. Chiropractors spend three or more years learning to skillfully adjust spinal vertebra. No other health provider even comes close to the depth of training and skill in spinal manipulation processed by the doctor of chiropractic.

Leg Length Discrepancy and Degeneration of the Spine, Hips, Knees and Joints of Foot and Ankle

As we have seen leg length discrepancy (LLD) is a major factor in the onset and progression of scoliosis but this is only the tip of the iceberg! Leg length inequality, where one leg is shorter than the other, represents the most significant factor in the development of osteoarthritis (OA) of the lower extremity and is a prime contributor to degeneration of the lumbar spine. LLD produces abnormal loading on the joints of our hips, legs and feet with an increase of approximately 6% of our body weight on the longer leg side![89] Out of sight and often undiagnosed, studies indicate that as many as 59% of the population has a difference in leg length of at least 5mm or more.[90] Often the difference is much greater.

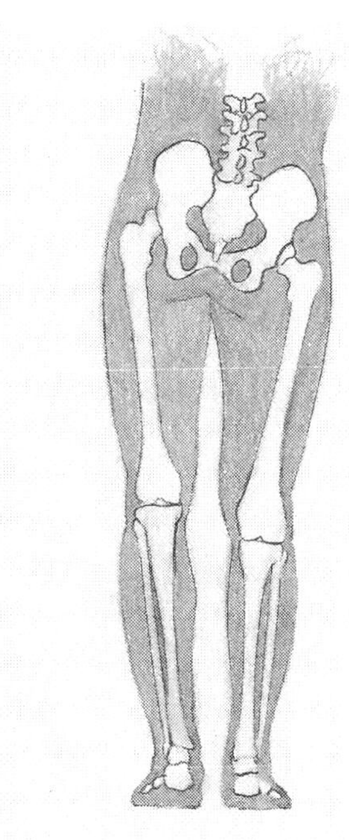

The skeleton may develop asymetrically producing leg length inequality.

Chronic joint pain, such as osteoarthritic degeneration of the hip, knee or lumbar spine has been estimated to affect 30% of the American population limiting the daily activities of approximately 50% of those affected.[91] In fact, low back pain, often associated with OA of the spinal joints and disc degeneration of the lumbar spine, is the most common cause of long-term disability in industrialized countries.[92]

So exactly how does a difference in leg length break down our joints? As you read earlier, leg length inequality creates an unlevel base for the spine. This action requires the flexible spine to shift or lean over the longer leg to balance the torso. This typically results in a functional or balancing spinal curve with its convexity toward the shorter leg. What goes unseen however, are the increased and abnormal pressures on the spinal discs, joints and vertebral bodies. Spinal structures on the concave side of curves must bear more weight leading to degeneration while ligaments encasing the spine are stretched on the convex side of curves. This can lead to shape malformations of the immature spine resulting in structural scoliosis. Secondarily, the pelvis composed of two large innominate bones on either side of the central sacrum subluxates as the innominate above the longer leg rotates backward while the innominate above the shorter leg side rotates forward! These rotations stress the large sacroiliac joints connecting the innominates to the sacrum and distort the movement patterns of the hip's ball and socket joints. These changes will eventually lead to OA of the hips and sacroiliac joints![93,94]

The body attempting to accommodate to the longer leg will often increase pronation or inward ankle deviation on the longer leg side as pronation flattens the foot effectively decreasing the height of the longer leg.[95] Abnormal pronation also creates an internal rotation of the knee when full weight is placed on the knee in walking. Inward deviation of the knee allows the lateral knee cap to rub against the 'U' shaped groove formed at the lower end of our upper leg bone or 'femur'. This wear can lead to softening and inflammation of the cartilage beneath the knee cap a condition known as 'chondromalacia patellae'. Pronation will also overstretch the anterior and posterior cruciate ligaments inside the knee leading to tears of these structures as well.[96,97]

As validation for these remarks, Golightly and colleagues looked at a random population of 926 men and women. They found that degeneration of the hip and knee was 80% higher in those with LLD.[98] Additionally, Friberg in a study of 547 Finnish Army conscripts involved in strenuous training and who had experienced stress fractures of the bones in their legs and feet found that 89% of the fractures occurred in those with an LLD of 3mm or more![99]

Radiologists seldom comment on leg length differences, even large differences. This is a huge disservice to the many pain sufferers who will never be adequately informed or treated correctly for their pain using lifted orthotic shoe inserts to regain their balance.

Spinal and Foraminal Stenosis

Spinal stenosis is a narrowing of the spinal canal and a brief overview of spinal anatomy is needed to understand this disorder. As we have seen the spine is made up of a series of connected bones (or vertebrae) and shock-absorbing discs between. Each vertebra contains a central round opening, formed in front by the main 'body' of the vertebrae which is joined by a rearward bony arch thereby encompassing the spinal cord and forming the spinal canal. Thus the spinal cord proper is encased in bone and travels from the brain downward inside each vertebra. At each joining of adjacent vertebra, the spinal cord gives off nerve roots emerging from either side to supply the organs of the body and direct their function. These nerves exit the spine through openings called the 'neural foramen'. The actual spinal 'cord' ends at the upper level of the lumbar spine, usually at the level of the first lumbar vertebra. Lumbar, sacral and coccygeal nerves emerge from the spinal cord's tip and descend down through the spinal canal to exit through the foramen of their respective vertebrae. This collection of nerves is termed the 'cauda equina', Latin for horse's tail which it roughly resembles. The cauda equina is also susceptible to compressive forces.

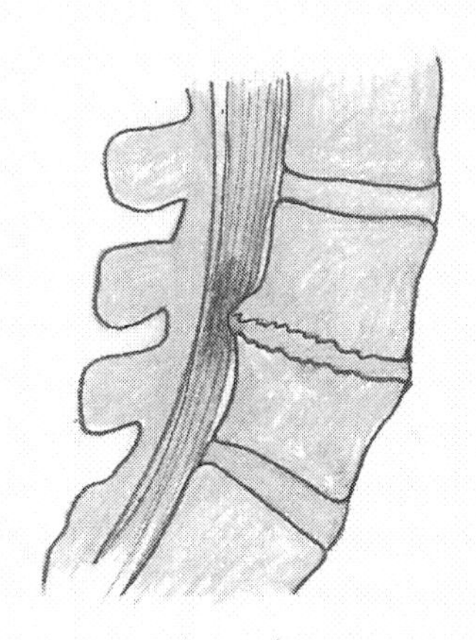

Lumbar stenosis due to old disc herniation and osteophyte formation

The spinal canal may be narrow from birth representing a congenital defect or acquired over time with aging, trauma or disc herniation. Spinal stenosis can therefore, occur at any age but is more likely to be encountered in seniors as wear and tear on the lumbar spine narrows the available space in the spinal canal. The leading reason for spinal stenosis is osteoarthritis, a condition caused by overloading the facets joints of the spine coupled with the breakdown of the disc cartilage which separates vertebra. Disc protrusion or herniation, thickening of spinal ligaments and calcified bone spurs secondary to spinal wear can further narrow the spinal canal. Compression can also occur following the excessive scarring associated with some spinal surgeries. (In rare cases tumor or disease processes affecting bone or neural tissue can also be responsible for cord and nerve compression.) Any combination of the above can produce pressure on the spinal cord or cauda equina. Unfortunately, individual nerves can be 'pinched' when neural foramen become reduced through the same mechanisms. (A process termed 'foraminal' or 'lateral recess' stenosis.)

Symptoms may vary from centralized back or neck pain or can be coupled with pain, numbing and weakness in the arms or torso but more often in the legs. Often with foraminal stenosis, individual nerves will be affected and nerve irritation can lead to 'neuropathy' or nerve pain like sciatica. If compression is severe walking can be difficult. A classic finding in lumbar spinal stenosis is the inability to walk for longer distances wherein the legs become heavy, numb and painful but a brief rest and bending relieve discomfort and allow further walking during which symptoms build again and require another bout of rest and bending. Severe spinal narrowing can affect the bowel, bladder and sexual function. More severe symptoms may present with atrophy or loss of muscle mass in the lower extremities and loss of neural control to the muscles of the legs and feet, resulting in foot-drop (causing one to 'slap' the foot on the ground while walking due to an inability to elevate the foot upward toward the shin).

Conservative medical approaches may include a variety of medications and may help in the short term but are not curative. Kinetic traction (reciprocal stretch and release traction methods available to many chiropractors) and chiropractic manipulation often bring short term relief due to their ability to mobilize and stretch the area, thereby increasing blood flow, decreasing restriction and altering compressive dynamics. Long term relief in severe cases involves surgical excision of compressive structures often with the removal of a portion of the posterior bony ring surrounding the rear of the spinal canal, thus allowing the spinal cord or cauda equina to have additional rearward space.

Spondylolisthesis

The word spondylolisthesis derives from two parts: spondylo, originating from ancient Greek, meaning spine or vertebra and listhesis,_or slippage. The term spondylolisthesis is used to indicate a forward slip of one vertebra relative to another. Spondylolisthesis usually occurs towards the base of the spine in the lumbar area. Commonly this condition originates due to fracture or congenital non-union of the posterior arch of the vertebra which would normally be attached to the vertebral body. Approximately

5%-6% of all males and 2%-3% of females have a spondylolisthesis. Physical endeavors such as weightlifting, gymnastics, soccer, football, etc. may precipitate spinal damage causing this condition and therefore the higher incidence in young males. 'Pratfalls', wherein one falls on ice with direct pelvic impact have long been recognized as a leading cause of spondylolisthesis as well.

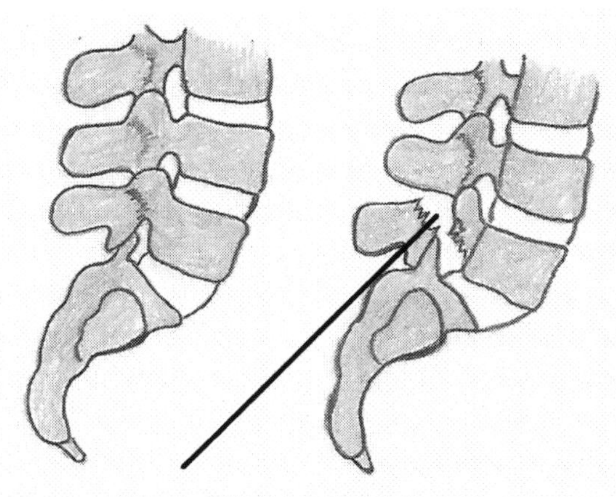

Spondylolestheisis

Displacement of a vertebra, relative to the vertebra below is not uncommon and may be seen in scoliosis or other spinal abnormalities. In such cases, terms like anterolisthesis, lateral listhesis or rotational listhesis may be used depending on the type of displacement. (Such abnormal spinal alignment may lead to asymmetric loads on the spine and spinal degeneration.)

Spondylolisthesis is graded according to its degree of severity, with a grade 1 being least advanced and grade 5 being most advanced. This grading is based on the location of the posterior body of the slipped vertebra relative to the body of the vertebra beneath it. Grading is fairly simple; on a lateral x-ray of the spine the top of the vertebral body below the slippage is divided into four equal parts. If the slipped vertebra above has moved slightly it is considered to be a grade one. If the back of the slipped vertebra is almost at the midpoint of the vertebra below (but not quite) it is graded as a two and so forth. If (in rare cases) the offending vertebra has slipped completely off the one below the slippage is graded as a five.

Usually, spondylolisthesis is only detected when back pain or injury dictates the need for diagnostic imaging. Symptoms that often accompany spondylolisthesis include:

Pain in the low back, especially after exercise
Increased lordosis (ie, swayback)
Pain and/or weakness in one or both thighs or legs
Reduced ability to control bowel and bladder functions
Tight hamstring musculature
Muscle spasms in the lower back

In cases of advanced spondylolisthesis, changes may occur in the way people stand and walk often demonstrating a waddling style of walking. This causes the abdomen to protrude further as the lower back curves forward more while the torso may seem shorter.

Most cases of spondylolisthesis are grades of one or two and are found in adult life having been likely present for years and may not be pain productive or unstable as the lower spine is well supported by strong muscles and retaining ligaments. Often, little needs to be done but it is advisable to avoid concussive activities like water skiing, skiing moguls or horseback riding. (Obesity definitely exacerbates this condition as it does in most spinal conditions.)

Spondylolisthesis initially identified with a grade of one or two should be monitored by x-ray no more than one year later to compare any progression of slippage. If none, then follow-up comparisons, can be of longer duration perhaps every two years or more baring any trauma to the lower back. Weight-bearing MRI's with flexion and extension are particularly good as an initial study to determine spinal stability. More significant grades of spinal slippage, especially those of three or greater, require a surgical consultation with an orthopedic or spine surgeon.

Ankylosis Spondylitis

Ankylosing spondylitis (AS) is an inflammatory disease, poorly understood and presently without a cure. Affecting more men than women, ankylosing spondylitis typically begins in early adulthood and over time causes calcified fusing of the spinal ligaments and vertebrae as well as connective tissue in other locations. These changes make the spine less flexible and can result in a hunched-forward posture. If spinal rib attachments are affected, it can be difficult to breathe deeply. AS typically begins in early adulthood initially affecting the spine. This condition can also impact sight with ocular redness, inflammation, pain, light sensitivity and blurred vision.

Early signs and symptoms of AS might include pain and stiffness in your lower back and hips, especially in the morning and after periods of inactivity. Neck pain and fatigue are also common. Over time, symptoms might worsen, improve or stop at irregular intervals.

The areas most commonly affected are:

The 'sacroiliac joints'; the joints between the sacrum at the base of the spine and the two large pelvic bones the 'innominates'

The vertebrae in your lower back, neck or tendon insertions at these locations

Tendons at the back of your heels

The cartilage between your breastbone and ribs

Your hip and shoulder joints

In severe ankylosing spondylitis, new bone forms as part of the body's attempt to heal. This new bone gradually bridges the gaps between vertebrae eventually fusing sections of the spine. Those areas become stiff and inflexible. Fusion can also stiffen your rib cage, restricting your lung capacity and function. Bone density can be lost during the early stages of AS weakening vertebrae which can collapse, increasing the severity of stooped posture which is common to this condition. Vertebral fractures can compress and possibly injure the spinal cord and nerves that pass through the spine. AS can also damage the aorta, the largest artery of the body carrying blood from the heart, as inflammation and enlargement distort the shape of the aortic heart valve impairing its function.

X-rays normally allow your doctor to check for changes in your joints and bones but the visible signs of ankylosing spondylitis may best be detected by MRI scans early in the disease process. AS has been associated with a gene known as HLA-B27. The vast majority of patients with ankylosing spondylitis have the gene but it is present in many individuals without this disorder.

The goal of treatment is to reduce inflammation, keep active and exercise in the early to mid-stages of the disease to maintain mobility and strength. Range-of-motion and stretching exercises can help maintain flexibility in your joints while proper sleep and walking positions coupled with abdominal and back exercises can help maintain your upright posture. Physical therapy or chiropractic spinal manipulation can be particularly helpful for many AS patients to ensure good spinal movement. Curcumin is the best choice for an anti-inflammatory in my opinion as NSAIDs, (like ibuprofen and naproxen sodium which are non-steroidal anti-inflammatories), reduce prostaglandins that are responsible for the manufacture of mucus secretions that coat our stomach and intestines. Long term usage of these NSAIDs can cause many problems, one of which is ulcerations as stomach acids burn the lining of the stomach and intestinal tract without this mucus coating.)

One of the simplest ways to ease inflammation associated with AS is to reduce your daily intake of 'Starchy Foods'. In 1996, a study was conducted in the UK by Alan Ebringer, M.D., who found that following a high-protein, low-starch diet could benefit people with ankylosing spondylitis. His further research published in 2006, demonstrated a strong link with bacterial overgrowth of Klebsiella pneumoniae in the digestive tracts of AS patients which when combined with the HLA-B27 gene (found in 96% of AS patients) is thought to produce the inflammatory changes seen in this condition.[100] Since Klebsiella pneumonia seems to thrive on diets heavy in simple carbohydrate consumption the low starch diet was suggested as a means to control the progression of the disease. In a clinical study, Finegold and coworkers carried out bacterial cultures on 47 vegetarian subjects on a high starch/low protein diet and compared these to 45 American subjects on an omnivorous diet involving low starch and high protein consumption. The mean number of Klebsiella microbes in the 'high starch' group was 30,000 bacteria per gram of feces compared to a value of 700 bacteria per gram of feces in those on a high protein diet.[101] Thus, it's no surprise that many AS patients have found the No Starch Diet beneficial. If you or a loved one has AS, check out the internet for the No Starch Diet for Ankylosing Spondylitis: What to Eat and Avoid.

For those experiencing ankylosis symptoms in the cervical spine, I would highly recommend the use of the Neck Correct or Curve Restorer exercise device as I have used this exercise tool with great success to decrease both pain and improve mobility in the cervical spines of many arthritic and ankylosing patients.

Plantar Fasciitis as a Biomechanical Problem

Lower heel pain, in that area contacting the ground, is typically due to either bruising of the 'calcaneus' or heel bone or to inflammation of the plantar tendons; two conditions quite different but often confused by health providers. Bruising the heel bone is common as with each step our weight is supported on a bone with less than a square inch of contact surface. Long hours of standing/walking barefoot or in non-supporting footwear can bruise the heel bone as can jogging and hard walking. While I have three beautiful daughters we could always tell when Jessie was about as we would hear her clumping around the house due to her heavy footsteps. Bruising of the heel is felt at the exact point of the lowest end of the heel bone, unlike plantar fasciitis (PF) which is felt slightly more forward toward the toes. Calcaneal bruising, unlike PF, is not typically associated with nerve pain.

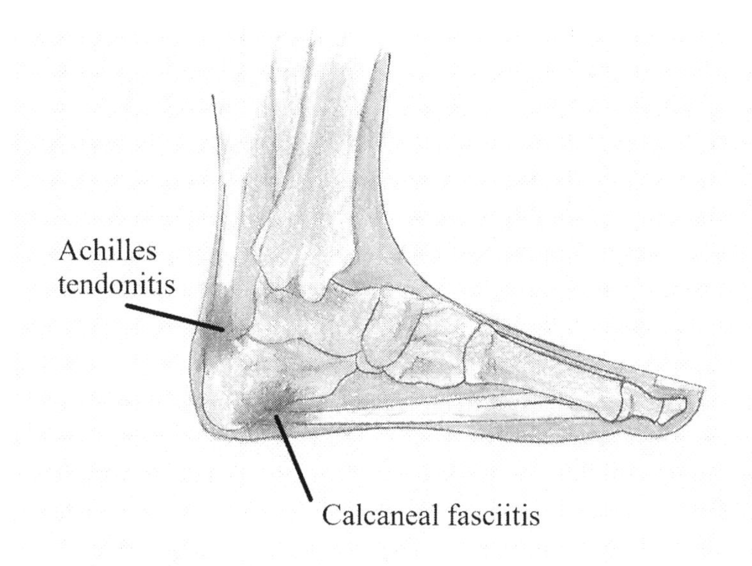

Plantar fasciitis results from damage to tendons that insert into the heel bone. Pain is felt on the underside of the foot about 2 inches (5 centimeters) forward from the back of the heel. PF may be associated with nerve pain affecting the bottom of the foot as well. Most patients with the diagnosis of plantar fasciitis are given a variety of stretches to perform or advised to use rollers or other devices to 'loosen' the connective tissue. Boots and other devices may also be employed to stretch the tendons by flexing the foot toward the shin. This is just nonsensical to me! Heel fasciitis involves micro-tearing and inflammation of the tendon fibers inserting into the heel. The last thing any logical person would wish to do is to further stretch the damaged tendon fibers already inflamed with micro-tears! Don't stretch or roll... read on.

Most often plantar fasciitis is connected to pronation (inward turning), of the ankle and foot! Each cycle of step sees the heel land in a normal and neutral position and then underweight to rock inward with pronation as the arch collapses. Thus there is a constant internal rotation of the calcaneus resulting in grinding of the plantar facial tendons with every step! Think of the old-time pharmacist as he takes his mortar and pestle and grinds the powders of his trade within his ceramic bowl! Just as he grinds his ingredients the heel grinds away at the plantar tendons inserting into the heel as it rolls in and out in an endless cycle of pronated gait!

As in other cases of soft tissue damage, ultrasound therapy, (usually done in a water bath due to the rounded contour of the heel), along with ice application, is the treatment of choice. Taking curcumin is recommended here as in all inflammatory conditions. Absolutely no massage, stretching or vibration should be done. Time and proper therapy assist resolution of the condition which often requires the formulation of quality shoe orthotics to balance the foot and to support and stabilize the arch in a neutral non-rocking position. If orthotics are needed, I will make light slip-off casts of the foot and send them to a podiatric lab with a prescription for the particulars of arch, padding, etc., needed in the appliance. Most chiropractors do not get this training which I received while in my study of orthopedics. A podiatrist is also a good choice for the fabrication of shoe inserts. Unfortunately, some podiatrists formulate such orthotics entirely from plastic. These plastic orthotics are often too uncomfortable to wear. A better choice is an orthotic with cushioning and possibly a sub-layer of material under the cushioned cover to provide a donut support for the outer rim of the heel and a slight pocket in which the inflamed tendon and bone may reside with less pressure while the orthotic use improves gait mechanics, lessens pain and improves the condition.

In some cases, long-standing irritation/inflammation of the ligaments attaching to the heel may result in a 'heel spur' or calcification which appears on x-ray as a spur or thorn-like projection from the heel. If sufficiently large surgery may be indicated.

Visit HealingTheHumanMachine.com for a video discussing this topic.

Metatarsalgia, Morton's Toe and Morton's Neuroma

Forefoot pain is a common condition especially affecting patients with a fondness for tight shoes or who have to stand for much of their day. This condition is often associated with a second toe that is longer than that of the first or large toe (Morton's toe). Here the second toe (or others) may be pushed backward in the shoe buckling the middle of the toe upward while pushing down on the base of the toe connected to the long bones of the foot known as the metatarsals. Prolonged overpressure in these areas can become exquisitely painful with swelling and arthritic changes in the ball of the foot. Electric or burning nerve pain may also be encountered in the later stages when delicate nerves between the toes become irritated often leading to Morton's neuroma. Larger shoes often coupled with custom orthotics are helpful as is therapeutic ultrasound done in a water bath. (Many people instinctively turn to massage or vibration to reduce forefoot pain. This is almost always a mistake and only prolongs the problem.)

Coccydynia (Coccyx Pain)

Patients presenting with coccyx pain are uncommon and primarily women who are five times more likely to develop this condition. Structural changes of the female pelvis required for childbearing render the female coccyx more exposed to injury. In addition, during the last trimester of pregnancy ligaments around this area soften to allow more movement of the pelvis for the birthing process. A baby's vaginal delivery can produce deflection of the coccyx which can strain any possible joints within its structure as well as surrounding tissue.

A more exposed coccyx will also make falls, especially 'prat' falls (where one lands directly on their derriere) more traumatic for women. Jarring activities like horseback or motorboat riding, prolonged sitting and certain sexual positions can also flair coccygeal pain. Uncommonly, infection or tumor may also cause painful symptoms and cannot be ruled out unless the onset of coccyx pain is linked to trauma.

Coccyx pain is seldom associated with displacement of the coccyx but more to bruising of tissue which in my experience responds beautifully to multiple sessions of ultrasound therapy. Special pillows with a U shaped cut out may be used to sit upon to alleviate coccyx pressure while sitting. As in other types of tissue inflammation manipulation of the area should be avoided unless x-ray demonstrates malposition.

Osteoarthritis

Osteoarthritis (OA), often termed 'wear and tear' arthritis, is by far the most common form of arthritis, affecting millions of people worldwide. It occurs when the protective cartilage that cushions the ends of our bones wears down over time due to physical stress and inflammation. Although osteoarthritis can damage any joint, this disorder most commonly affects joints in your hands, knees, hips and spine.

Osteoarthritis symptoms often develop slowly and worsen over time as mechanical stresses on the joints take their inevitable toll. Signs and symptoms of osteoarthritis include:

Pain in the joints during or after movement

Joint stiffness most noticeable upon awakening or after being inactive

Tenderness when you apply light pressure to or near the joint

Loss of flexibility and limited range of motion

A grating sensation like sand in the joint or popping or crackling on movement

Bone spurs presenting as hard lumps found around the affected joint

Swelling caused by soft tissue inflammation in the joint

According to the Mayo Clinic factors that can increase your risk of osteoarthritis include: old age, sex (women seem to have a higher incidence), genetics, metabolic diseases, joint injuries, excess weight and finally repeated stress to the joint. In my experience, this last factor is by far the major contributor to OA in that faulty body mechanics will wear the joint over time.

Joints are richly endowed with protective cartilage that covers bone ends. These tough cartilaginous pads are well lubricated by 'synovial fluid', a slippery substance secreted by non-weight bearing tissues in the joints that ease and enhance joint movement. Further the joint is stabilized by very strong ligaments and muscles to maintain proper alignment in movement. When normal movement patterns are disrupted a gradual disintegration of the joint begins to occur as retaining ligaments become stretched and damaged joint tissues become inflamed. Inflammation decreases the 'oily' viscosity or lubrication of the synovial fluid as friction builds in the joints degrading them. Eventually, the cartilage that protects bone ends becomes so swollen and inflamed that pieces of the cartilage break apart, thin, calcify and erode leaving the bone ends with little or no padding, protection or lubrication. Loss of cartilage in the joint acts in a similar fashion as loss of disc height in the spine, allowing the bone ends to have more play or motion within the joint. Overtime, excess motion within the joint leads to erosion of the bone surfaces themselves and development of bone spurs (thorn-like projections from the margins of joints) where ligaments attach due to repeated tugging from excess joint motion.

The bottom line; time and use unavoidably wears our human machine but if you have persistent joint pain get your alignment checked by a competent body mechanic; a chiropractor.

Forward Head Posture, the Most Common Reason for Chronic Neck Pain and Degeneration

Imagine holding a twelve-pound bowling ball balanced directly above your elbow rested on a table. Not so difficult is it? Now move the bowling ball forward and inch and hold it for a minute. Now move the bowling ball forward another inch and hold it for a minute. Getting harder? Now move it forward another inch and the muscles in your forearm begin to ache. Well, this is exactly what is happening to the muscles of the neck and upper back as a straightened or often reversed cervical curve projects your head forward and out of balance with your body, a condition known as forward head posture (FHP). Forward head posture, is the most common abnormal body posture and occurs when the head is positioned anterior or forward of a vertical line which should pass through the ear canal of the erect head to descent through the mid-point of the erect shoulder and downward intersecting the mid-hip and leg.

As you've read, for every inch of forward head position, the weight of the head doubles, then triples, etc., as the muscles of the neck and upper back have to work ever harder to hold the head from toppling forward. This singular biomechanical distortion leads to an entire constellation of health complications as diverse as faulty balance and vertigo to depression and sexual dysfunction. Forward head posture's roll in chronic neck and upper back pain has been well documented.[102,103,104,105]

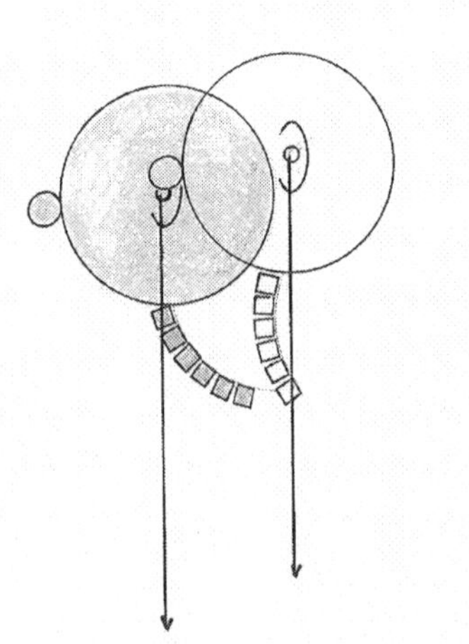

Forward head posture
magnifies muscular load.

FHP abnormally loads the joints and discs of the cervical spine increasing the compression forces on these spinal structures resulting in their early decay. According to Dr. A. I. Kapandji, who authored the prestigious 'Physiology of the Joints', forward head translation also places constant pressure on the large occipital nerves that emerge from the base of the skull encircling our scalp playing a role in occipital neuralgia. Researchers have also found troubling connections between forward head posture and TMJ, migraine, carpal tunnel, stroke, and falling in the elderly. FHP can lead to shoulder impingement, thoracic outlet syndrome, obstructive sleep apnea, hearing loss, thoracic kyphosis and the progression to 'Dowager's Hump', low back pain, fibromyalgia and impaired blood flow to the brain.[106, 107, 108, 109, 110, 111, 112, 113, 114, 115, 116, 117, 118, 119, 120, 121]

Forward head posture

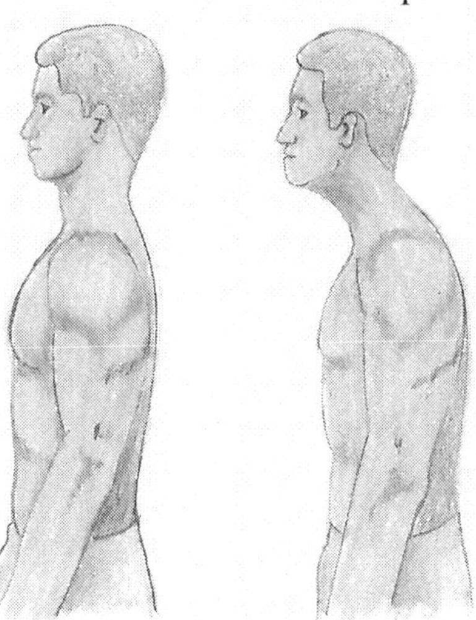

How do we acquire FHC? Stomach sleeping and traumas like falls or motor vehicle accidents certainly are responsible to some degree but today in our heavy computer and cell phone dependent world we accelerate the process by spending countless hours with our necks flexed downward! As a result, we have even adopted the new terminology of 'text neck' and 'turtle neck syndrome' as in a prolonged neck flexed position we radically change the architecture of our spine!

Visit HealingTheHumanMachine.com for a video discussing forward head posture.

Forward Head Posture and TMJ Disorder

Earlier we touched on TMJ briefly but it deserves a bit more attention since it's estimated that 12% of us have this disorder. To be sure, structural abnormalities of the jaw joint can be a factor but many TMJ sufferers have normal jaw structure. So why TMJ? Numerous studies point to forward head posture (FHP) as a prime factor! Forward head posture most commonly presents as an elongation and straightening of the lower cervical spine and often a more curved upper cervical spine. This abnormal posture distorts jaw movement and tightens jaw muscles stressing the TMJ. As with any untreated bio-mechanical stress, faulty movement patterns wreak havoc over time.

What to do? Get a better curve in your cervical spine. How? Stop stomach sleeping, elevate your laptops, monitors and text devices to keep your head more erect and start to exercise. Daily Neck Correct exercises can dramatically reduce forward head posture but the fix is not fast taking usually six to twelve months of diligent use.

If you've been diagnosed with TMJ but have normal jaw structure, most often the case in those whose jaw doesn't pop and click with chewing, chew gum. Gum chewing is ill-advised if you have a significant structural problem of the jaw joint but if FHP is the sole mechanism for your TMJ there is no reason not to give the jaw muscles a little extra exercise. Contrary to the advice of many gurus, it has been my clinical experience that you need to stretch tightened jaw muscles.

The Curve Restorer 'Neck Correct'

Correction of forward head posture (FHP) is paramount and indelibly associated with the straightening or reversal of the cervical spine. Many years ago, when faced with treating this problem I was presented with a limited array of options and devices. Most of these seemed frankly barbaric and some possibly injurious. Many employed weights hanging off head-straps or sling devices that seemed more akin to torture than therapy. These devices were primarily stretching reversed curves but incorporated either no or only static muscular work. I felt an effective device must allow for a combination of both stretch and muscle strengthening exercises.

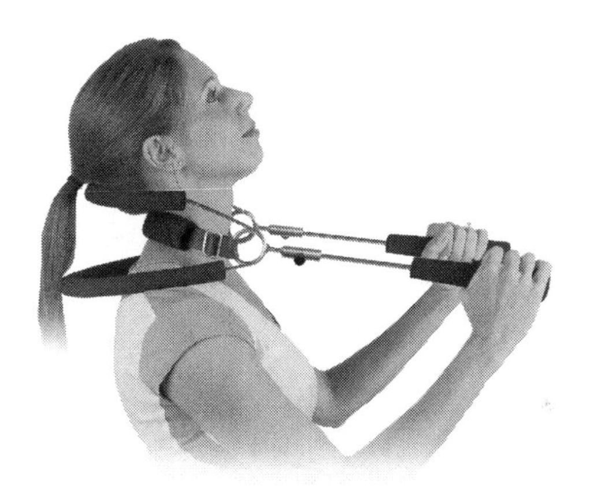

Sitting down at the drawing board I began to envision a device that could simultaneously stretch a kyphotic cervical curve into a more normal position and then work the muscles of the neck and upper back to strengthen and hold the newly forming lordotic curve. Thus, over time and with many renditions the 'Curve Restorer' (AKA Neck Correct) was born and is a popular device to relieve neck pain and assist cervical spine rehabilitation. The device is simplicity itself. As the unit is drawn into the rear neck a padded upper loop rests lightly on the rearward skull and a lower contoured area rests on the upper shoulders. Simultaneously an elastic strap is drawn into the mid-neck stretching the spine forward to achieve a more forward or normal lordotic spinal curve.

With the spinal curve held in a better position a series of exercises are begun as the head is extended backward against the force of spring steel coils attached to the arms of the loops. As extension maneuvers become easier additional exercises can be added to work not only the posterior spinal muscles but also the lateral and frontal neck musculature as well. The exercises are only mildly strenuous and can be accomplished by even those individuals who are somewhat frail as they begin to do a minimal number of repetitions and increase them accordingly as their strength and flexibility are restored.

The unit was designed initially to re-balance the head and improve spinal curvature and has demonstrated great effectiveness in that regard. In addition to curve restoration, the Neck Correct is an excellent rehab tool to relax overworked and fatigued neck and upper back muscles after a long day of computer work and to strengthen those areas post-injury. Those with arthritic necks, radicular (nerve) pain or considering spinal surgery often find relief and increased mobility with the exercises and some have canceled scheduled surgeries during its use.

Like all exercise equipment, the Curve Restorer or Neck Correct should be used judiciously. Exercises should begin slowly and with just a few repetitions to gauge the user's response, gradually increasing the number of exercises and repetitions performed over time. Those with acute or severe neck pain should avoid its use until their pain is reduced through proper therapy. If any adverse effects should be encountered, use of the device should be discontinued and a knowledgeable health care practitioner consulted.

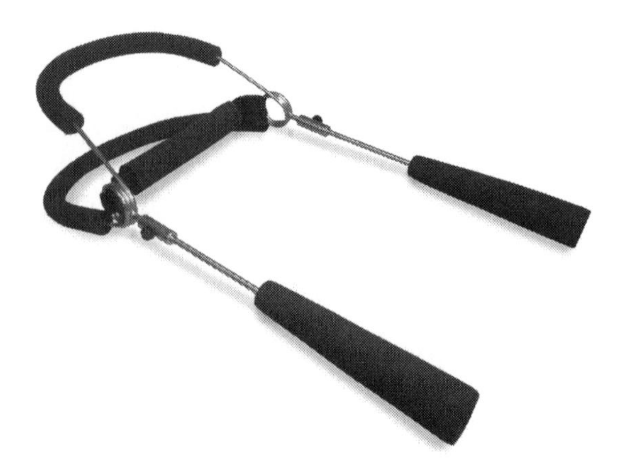

The Neck Correct can be purchased by visiting HealingTheHumanMachine.com.

Where Do Headaches Come From?

Those with an active headache disorder comprise roughly 46% of the global population.[122] There are three broad categories of headaches; cervicogenic headaches coming from the neck, tension headaches also coming from muscular structures of the neck typically and the rest about 17% migraine headaches.[123] In light of our previous discussion on forward head posture (FHP) we can easily understand that cervicogenic and tension headaches can easily be caused by the excessive strain related to carrying the head forward in an unbalanced position. In fact, researchers found in a study of 47 individuals with tension-type headaches and migraines that 77% of the subjects had a marked reduction in the normal forward (lordotic) cervical spine curvature or an outright reversal of the curve.[124] This in turn, places great stress on the individual joints in the cervical spine producing disrupted and restricted movement patterns of individual cervical vertebrae. Increased load or aberrant movement patterns in the spinal joints of the neck have been shown in numerous studies to cause headaches and is the reason that so many headache victims respond well to chiropractic adjustments of spinal vertebrae.[125,126]

Migraine headaches are a bit more of an enigma however and many differing opinions have prevailed as to causation. Since the brain itself has no pain receptors it feels no pain. However the outer coverings of our brain, the 'meninges' are richly supplied with pain nerves as is the scalp and the outer covering of the skull just below the scalp known as the ‘periosteum’. Some researchers have held fast to the belief that migraines are primarily a higher brain (cerebral) event, often vascular in nature, wherein blood vessels located in the brain and just beneath the meninges may release toxic chemicals irritating their pain receptors. Today migraine etiology is finally being clarified and points to a very small region of the brain, the 'brainstem'.

Like a turnip, the brain has a stem at its base and that stem is larger as it exits narrowing down toward the tip of the root. Similarly, the brainstem is larger as it emerges from the brain narrowing as it passes downward through the base of the skull via a circular opening known as the 'foramen magnum' and into the upper two cervical vertebrae. These upper vertebrae, the atlas and axis, have a larger internal diameter than the vertebrae below them to accommodate the lowest part of the brainstem, the 'medulla'. At the level of the third cervical vertebra the brainstem medulla narrows somewhat to become the spinal cord proper which is reflected in the reduced inner diameter of the third cervical vertebra.[127]

Sophisticated imaging using positron emission tomography or PET scans that can access brain physiology in real-time have demonstrated that prior to, during and after a migraine the brainstem is activated before and long after other areas of the brain have normalized.[128] Pulling vast amounts of research together, Dr. J. Tajti and colleagues in their paper 'Where does a migraine attack originate? In the brainstem.', clearly demonstrate the brainstem as the generator of migraines as disturbance here sets off a cascade of upper brain 'depolarization' and vascular disturbance.[129] Other researchers have linked the brainstem to the nausea, light and sound intolerance of migraine.[130,131]

Although small in size the brainstem medulla may be considered one of the most important parts of the brain as it controls and influences myriad functions that support and sustain life. It is here that our automatic and unthinking control centers reside for important functions like breathing, blood pressure, heartbeat regulation and gastrointestinal function but that's just the tip of the iceberg. Descending into the brainstem are many individual nerve tracts from higher brain centers for communication and regulation with and by the brainstem. As a result, the brainstem also influences the sense of taste, swallowing, speech, saliva production, balance and eye movements, nausea, vomiting, sleep state and arousal, fine touch, pressure sense and information about body part position and load, blood vessel dilation and constriction, sexual function and orgasm, motor function to the limbs, coordination and even mood; anxiety and depression have been linked to neurotransmitters secreted and influenced by the brainstem![132,133,134,135] Another finding of great interest to those suffering from fibromyalgia, is that the brainstem is largely responsible for determining how much physical pain we feel and injury or pain in distant areas of the body can make the brainstem more sensitive to pain to the extent that even non-painful touch causes pain.[136,137,138]

The importance of the anatomical position of the brainstem is profound. Encased in a rigid skull there is little that can affect the brain but encasing the lowest portion of the brainstem in the upper two cervical vertebrae is a whole different matter! Numerous studies have indicated that brainstem pressure by the atlas and axis can result in pain and dysfunction in many areas of the body.[139] As David Butler states in his book 'The Sensitive Nervous System', the brain effectively floats in the cerebrospinal fluid and moves in synchrony with the skull, receiving the odd bumps on the head that everyone gets. For this, the brain is well protected by its cranial cushioning or 'meninges' and the skull. However, head movement has a significant mechanical effect on the brainstem; when the head and spine are moved, the shape of the brainstem and spinal cord changes. The brainstem can be stretched a centimeter and a half longer form cervical spine extension to flexion. In flexion, upper brain cranial nerves are pulled tight at their exit zones in the medulla at the base of the skull as is the medulla itself.[140,141] Flexion also increases the angle between the upper spine and the medulla effectively pulling the medulla into the bony frontal edges of the axis, atlas and foramen magnum while simultaneously stretching the brainstem thus magnifying frontal pressure on the brain stem.[142]

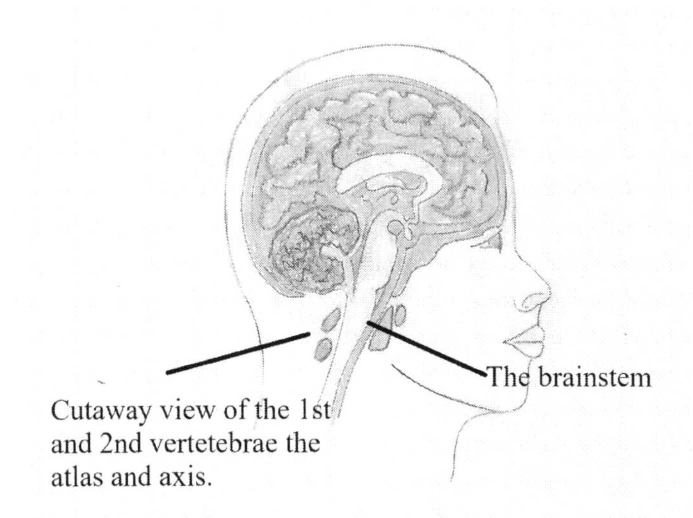
The brainstem
Cutaway view of the 1st
and 2nd vertetebrae the
atlas and axis.

What does all this mean? When we flex our necks downward or when we have cervical curve reversal often found with forward head posture we stretch the upper cervical spinal cord downward, pulling the brainstem downward as well. Since the brainstem is sized to fit into the atlas and axis but not the third cervical vertebrae this represents a 'tight squeeze' as it moves slightly downward and against surrounding bony elements of the spine and skull. Could the simple act or having a reversed cervical curve cause enough brainstem irritation to impact a host of health problems? An interesting study appearing in the 2007 Journal of Human Hypertension, provides some food for thought; fifty patients with high blood pressure had a lowering of their blood pressure with chiropractic adjustments of the atlas to reduce brainstem pressure with results similar to a two-drug combination therapy![143] In another study sixty-seven patients with staggering and balance issues were evaluated before and just after having cervical spine manipulations with marked improvement in balance after their adjustment.[144] In a third study with migraine sufferers, one hundred and twenty-seven individuals with migraine were divided into two groups; forty received no treatment and were used as controls while eighty-seven received two months of chiropractic cervical spine manipulation not exceeding sixteen treatments. Eighty-three of the eighty-seven had significant reductions in headache frequency, duration, disability and medication use following the chiropractic care.[145]

So let's take a moment and consider what the effects might be if those with balance disorders, headaches, visual or hearing problems, nausea, fibromyalgia, insomnia, sexual dysfunction, swallowing or speaking difficulty, incoordination, hypertension, taste affectation, or other conditions received chiropractic spinal adjustments to the atlas and axis, the two uppermost spinal vertebrae? Might there be an improvement in any number of conditions? And even if the brainstem were only a minor contributor to such conditions, which research is showing it is clearly not, wouldn't even slight improvement with a low risk, non-drug therapy like chiropractic manipulation be a good idea?

The Mismanagement of Scoliosis

The conventional treatment of spinal scoliosis by the medical profession has not changed much in the last 70 years. Usually, those with scoliotic curves are monitored for curve progression. If curvatures increase dramatically, bracing or spinal surgery is employed.

If one looks at scoliosis causation, one will find that a small number of scoliosis cases are due to congenital or neuromuscular conditions. The majority of scoliosis cases however, approximately 80%, are classified as 'idiopathic' or of unknown cause. It is stunning in the present day to have a condition so prevalent with so few answers. Some of the reasons for the mystery surrounding scoliosis are both surprising and disturbing! Before we discuss some of the roots of this confusion let me share with you my personal experience.

In the early days of my practice, I began seeing children and adults with scoliosis. Often I was the first person to have ever given them the diagnosis as the routine examination of children to detect abnormal spinal curvatures is usually done by school nurses, gym teachers or pediatricians who are often not very good at this. In other cases, when I reviewed spinal x-rays which had previously been ordered by other doctors, I was routinely seeing 'collimated' x-rays, (x-rays limited to the flexible spine without including the pelvis and upper legs). As I began to evaluate and measure the numerous discrepancies seen on a proper scoliosis x-ray study, (one that views the lumbar spine, entire pelvis and upper femurs where our legs connect to the hip sockets), it became very obvious that the vast majority of scoliosis patients I was encountering had a very concrete reason for abnormal spinal curvature. Their scoliosis was caused by a spine attempting to balance itself atop an unlevel base! An unlevel base caused by a difference in leg length or less commonly due to structural malformations of the pelvis or lower spine.

It was when I began to compare the radiology reports with the actual x-ray films of scoliosis studies performed outside my office that I was completely flabbergasted! X-ray studies revealing the presence of a short leg or other pelvic abnormality creating an unlevel platform or base for the flexible spine were never mentioned in the radiologist's reports! Imagine looking at the x-ray of an eight-year-old with a scoliotic lumbar curvature and never mentioning that one leg was 1/2 inch shorter than the other; a discrepancy producing a tilted base for the spine to rest on! Since pediatricians were not looking at the actual x-rays, (as they are not usually trained to read x-rays films), they were depending solely on the radiologist's report! So if a leg length discrepancy was seen by the radiologist, but without his or her comment in the x-ray report, the pediatrician would never know of the presence of a difference in leg length! In my opinion, the reason that the medical community continues to regard the majority of scoliosis cases as idiopathic has much to do with this single and (in my experience) nearly universal omission of reporting by medical radiologists!

An interesting study was published in the July 2010 edition of the Archives of Medical Science.[146] A group of researchers had noted the high correlation between leg length difference and scoliosis. They determined that children with one leg shorter than the other caused a lowering of the pelvis on the deficient (lower leg) side resulting in lumbar scoliosis with curvature usually towards the shorter extremity. They also found that as many as 15% of the population had a leg length difference (LLD)! (Other studies have found a much higher incidence of LLD as was noted earlier.) Between 1998 and 2006, children aged 5 to 17 years with LLD related scoliosis were treated with a shoe lift for the short leg side. Among 369 children the discrepancy of 0.5 cm was observed in 27, 1 cm in 329, 1.5 cm in 9 and 2 cm in 4 children. Each of the children were given shoe lifts to equalize leg length. During the first follow-up examination and within 2 weeks, adjustment of the spine to the shoe lifts was noted and correction of the curves occurred in 316 (or 83.7%) of the examined children! In 53 children (14.7%) the correction was observed later and was accompanied by slight low back pain. Leg length discrepancy equalization with shoe lifts had resulted in the elimination of scoliosis in almost all of the cases!

Let's imagine however that these researchers had not corrected the scoliotic curves. Body balance is important and without it we would have difficulty functioning. The Tower of Pizza tilts because its foundation is unlevel but children are not buildings and must balance themselves to operate efficiently. A child with a short leg leans their torso toward the upper or longer leg side to maintain balance. This creates a curve in the spine. Initially, this curve is a 'balancing or functional curve' whose vertebrae remain normal in shape. Soon however things may begin to change. In a groundbreaking study published in the March 1993 edition of 'Spine', researchers demonstrated conclusively that the worsening of scoliotic curvatures was the result of unequal forces acting on the immature bone.[147] "Osseous growth was disturbed in the scoliotic curve, the vertebra became deformed, and the vertebral body became wedge-shaped. Spinal vertebrae, still soft and transitioning from cartilage to bone in the immature spine and under pressure on the concave sides of the spinal curves slowed their growth and became deformed in shape turning functional scoliosis into structural scoliosis!

This is an important and fundamental concept in the progression of scoliosis as a 'balancing curve' secondary to an unleveling of the spine or pelvis will, through compressional and traction effects, succumb to morphological or shape changes of the vertebrae over time. Vertebrae on the concave side of a balancing curve are subject to compression forces while vertebrae on the convex side are subject to traction effects. Thus vertebrae in an abnormal curve formation are subject to both compression and traction! In support of this fact, Ian Stokes and a team of researchers applied surgical implants to rat tail vertebrae capable of either compression or traction to the immature vertebrae. Loaded (compressed) vertebrae grew at only 68% of non-loaded vertebrae and tractioned (stretched) vertebrae grew 114% longer than the non-tractioned vertebrae![148] Aronsson, et al., duplicated these studies finding compressed vertebrae achieved only 68% of the height of non-compressed vertebrae and tractioned vertebrae elongated 123% more than non-stretched controls! And all of this in just six weeks![149] In 1998 these researchers further demonstrated that such forces had the same effects on spinal discs![150]

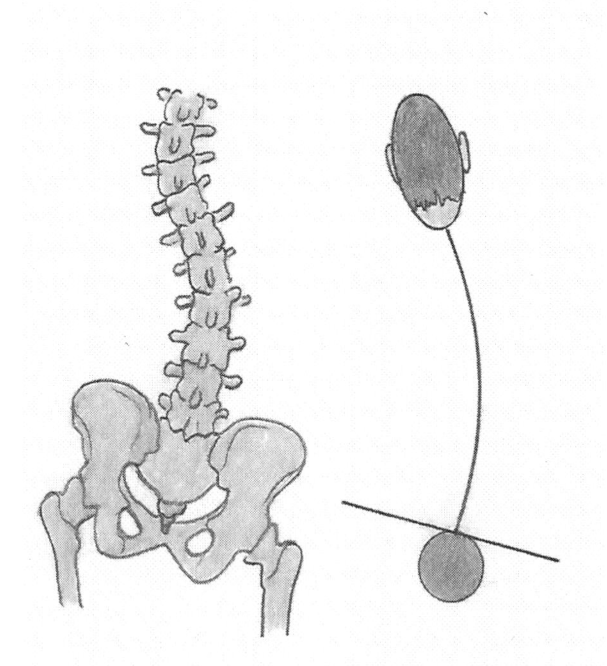

The spine attempts to balance itself.

Over many years of practice, I have performed thousands of spinal x-ray studies and many of these were for scoliosis. In that time I have encountered relatively few scoliosis cases that were not the result of a leg length difference or other unleveling spinal influence. The flexible spine with its 24 movable vertebrae is a 'teeter-totter' that is balanced on the pelvis. Anything that imbalances the pelvis will produce a 'compensatory' spinal curve above as the body attempts to re-balance itself. A left leg that is one-half inch shorter than the right leg will usually result in a compensatory convex curve of the thoracic (mid-back) or lumbar (low back) spinal region toward the lower left side as the weight of the torso is shifted to the higher side. As we have seen, leg length differences are common. Equally common are structural developmental abnormalities of the pelvis, sacrum or lower lumbar vertebrae that produce unleveling of the spine above. It is estimated that between 6 and 9 percent of the population have scoliosis! Given that a high percentage of us have a short leg I think the correlation is pretty clear.

One can see that in the treatment of scoliosis that full view, non-collimated x-ray studies are important and radiologists must begin to universally report instances of leg length discrepancy or other findings of pelvic or spinal inequality. As we have seen vertebral deformity due to abnormal pressures can happen quickly. When it comes to children diagnosed with scoliosis the clock is always ticking and expedient, knowledgeable treatment is extremely important.

Visit HealingTheHumanMachine.com for a video discussing scoliosis.

Suspect Scoliosis? How to do a Home Exam

If you are questioning whether you or your child may have scoliosis the first thing to do is take a good look at your child or have someone take a good look at you. Removing exterior clothing is a must. The observer must look for good body conformation as they stand behind the individual in question. Stance and posture during the exam are important and the person suspected of having scoliosis should stand erect and with their feet placed directly under the hips. (It should be understood that the hips are actually an inch or more inside the body's outer width depending on body mass.) For most adults, the distance between the feet should be 12 inches and both feet should be on an imaginary line parallel to the wall in front of them. For younger children, this distance may be 8 to 10 inches depending on size. Look for overall good posture and particularly look at the apparent levelness of the lower back. Does one hip seem higher? Feel the back and large pelvic bones. Kneeling behind the subject and placing one's hands on the top of the pelvic bones is one way to judge. Look at shoulder height as well realizing that hand dominance usually produces a slight drop in shoulder height on the corresponding side which is normal. (A right-hand dominant individual would be highly suspect for scoliosis if they demonstrated a high right shoulder for instance.) Look at the torso and divide the two sides with the spinal depression as the midline. Do both sides seem equally divided? Does one side seem wider or more highly developed and if so is this area more prominent or does it seem posterior as compared to the adjacent side? Is there an abnormal crease on one side of the lower back absent from the other side? Look at the feet again. Do the feet and pelvis face the wall but the shoulders rotate left or right a few degrees? Does the head sit squarely atop the torso without tilt? A tilted head or rotated torso out of balance with the pelvis is another strong indicator of potential scoliosis. Holding the patient's hips, have them bend forward ninety degrees. Sighting along the back of the bent-over individual, do both sides of the torso appear level or is one area elevated? Elevation on one side is a further indicator of scoliosis. The bottom line: take a good look and don't trust your pediatrician, school nurse or gym coach to do the looking for you or to necessarily know what they're looking at if they do!

If you or your child has been diagnosed or is suspected of having scoliosis it is paramount to receive a quality x-ray study (always done standing), with the inclusion of the femur heads (top of the leg bones) on the study. You should speak with the radiologist reading the study (or orthopedist in some cases) and ask them directly if they see any discrepancy in leg length or any other bony abnormality of the lower spine or pelvis that could unlevel the spine. If they indicate yes or equivocate take the actual films to a spinal expert; a chiropractor or chiropractic specialist.

Since many cases of scoliosis begin as compensatory curves in the beginning, early intervention is best. Often an orthotic shoe insert to elevate the shorter leg coupled with spinal manipulation and specific rehabilitation exercises or other techniques employed by a knowledgeable chiropractor or chiropractic specialist can put things right in the shortest amount of time. Even in advanced cases these and other procedures performed by a knowledgeable health provider can be extremely beneficial to arrest or improve spinal curvatures.

Reading Your Spinal X-rays...A Limited Interpretation

Medical radiologists have excellent training in identifying pathologies like cancer, joint degeneration, fracture, disc pathology and many other abnormalities of the human body. Their training in this regard is truly first-rate. They have however, little understanding or appreciation of spinal biomechanics. When the medical radiologist looks at spinal x-rays he or she is looking for pathology vs. normality. When the chiropractor looks at spinal x-rays they look for pathology as well but also evaluate structural abnormalities that create abnormal spinal mechanics. This careful analysis allows them to formulate a method of conservative treatment and correction!

While I read the radiologist's reports, I also evaluate these studies as well, requesting copies of films when performed outside my office. Often these reports fail to identify or correctly address the importance of the most basic mechanical problems of the spine. It's one thing to identify arthritic joints but even more important to identify the abnormal spinal stresses creating arthritis! Radiologists routinely and incorrectly blame abnormal spinal curvatures like cervical kyphosis and forward head posture on spasm or faulty positioning by x-ray techs during exams! The mention of spinal unleveling due to leg length or pelvic deficiencies is rarely mentioned. Information concerning lumbar spinous and facet compression, lumbar lordosis or thoracic kyphosis are typically missing from radiology reports! These and a myriad of other omissions are a terrible misfortune for spinal pain patients because these neglected abnormalities are responsible for much of their suffering.

This lack of reporting is extremely profound because if you cannot or do not identify a problem you can't fix it! Spinal abnormalities revealed on weight-bearing x-rays can pinpoint the cause of spinal pain and degeneration providing the vital information needed to correct those mechanical and structural faults. Proper x-ray evaluation is critical to choosing the palliative and healing therapies, specific rehab exercises or orthotic appliances needed to correct or minimize spinal pain or referred nerve pain like sciatica. If you've ever seen an engineer look at blueprints this is the same scrutiny given to spinal x-rays by chiropractors and speaks to the extensive training that is drilled into the brains of aspiring young chiropractic students over two or more years as they spend long hours in classrooms visualizing thousands of x-ray, MRI and CT scans!

The largest single misconception by the general public is that M.D.s are superior to chiropractors in treating musculoskeletal and particularly spinal pain. Nothing is further from the truth! Beginning with an often incomplete evaluation and report of your spinal x-rays by the medical radiologist, the problem is further compounded when the report is then sent to your M.D. who seldom sees these studies and has limited training in the treatment of musculoskeletal conditions. M.D. care of spinal pain can therefore be ineffective at best and often leads to needless testing, incorrect therapy and prolonged pain!

One might think that the orthopedist or pain specialist would be a good resource to turn to but this choice can be equally wrong. Pain specialists are great at giving more and specialized pain control measures and orthopedists are trained to do surgery but in most cases neither group knows much about the engineering analysis of weight-bearing spinal x-rays or the conservative measures to treat and correct the spinal defects revealed by such analysis. That could be why low back pain is the number one workplace injury accounting for more cost and lost productivity than any other condition or the reason why only 18% of chronic pain patients ever get better. Medical intervention is also a contributing factor to our epidemic of opioid and other forms of drug abuse in this country.[151] In the next few pages we'll look at some x-rays of my patients and the actual medical radiologist's report of findings. Each will be followed by my evaluation. It should be very interesting.

NAME:MATTHEWS,KEVIN
MRN: 8026648
DOB: 10/4/2002, Sex: M
Acct #: 50171580052
ARRIVAL: 6/7/2017, D/C: 6/7/2017

***** Final result *****

Ordering Provider:	Calvin Hargis, DC	*Authorizing Provider:*	Calvin Hargis, DC
Ordering Phone:	845-986-5500	*Authorizing Phone:*	
Ordering Fax:	845-986-6627	*Attending Provider:*	
Ordering Pager:		*PCP:*	

Other Ordering Provider:

Procedure:	**XR SPINE LUMB 2 OR 3 V [72100]**
Procedure Date:	06/07/2017 10:20 AM
Accession Number:	103352436
Order Number:	387438921
Ordering Diagnosis:	Lumbalgia [M54.5 (ICD-10-CM)]
Reason for Exam:	Lumbalgia
Performing Department:	DEPARTMENT
Patient Class:	OUTPATIENT

Study Result

Radiographs of the lumbar spine

performed on 6/7/2017 10:00 AM

for patient
male of 14 years

CLINICAL INFORMATION: Lumbalgia

TECHNIQUE: Frontal and lateral views of the lumbar spine and lateral coned-down view of the lumbosacral junction were obtained.

FINDINGS: No previous examinations are available for review.

Patient is skeletally immature. Patient is leaning to the LEFT Lumbar vertebral alignment is maintained. Lumbar vertebral body heights are preserved. Pedicles are intact. No fracture or destructive bone lesions are seen.

Lumbar intervertebral disc spaces appear intact. Disc heights are maintained. No significant productive changes are found.

The sacroiliac joints appear intact.

IMPRESSION
IMPRESSION: Unremarkable radiographs of the lumbar spine.

THIS DOCUMENT HAS BEEN ELECTRONICALLY SIGNED BY MD

Result History

XR SPINE LUMB 2 OR 3 V (Order #387438921) on 6/7/2017 - Order Result History Report

This is the medical radiologist's report of the weight-bearing or standing x-ray views of my patient Kevin Matthews, a fourteen-year-old male. It is interesting to note that this study was read as normal and the radiologist who was not present when the technologist performed the study states that Kevin was leaning to the left.

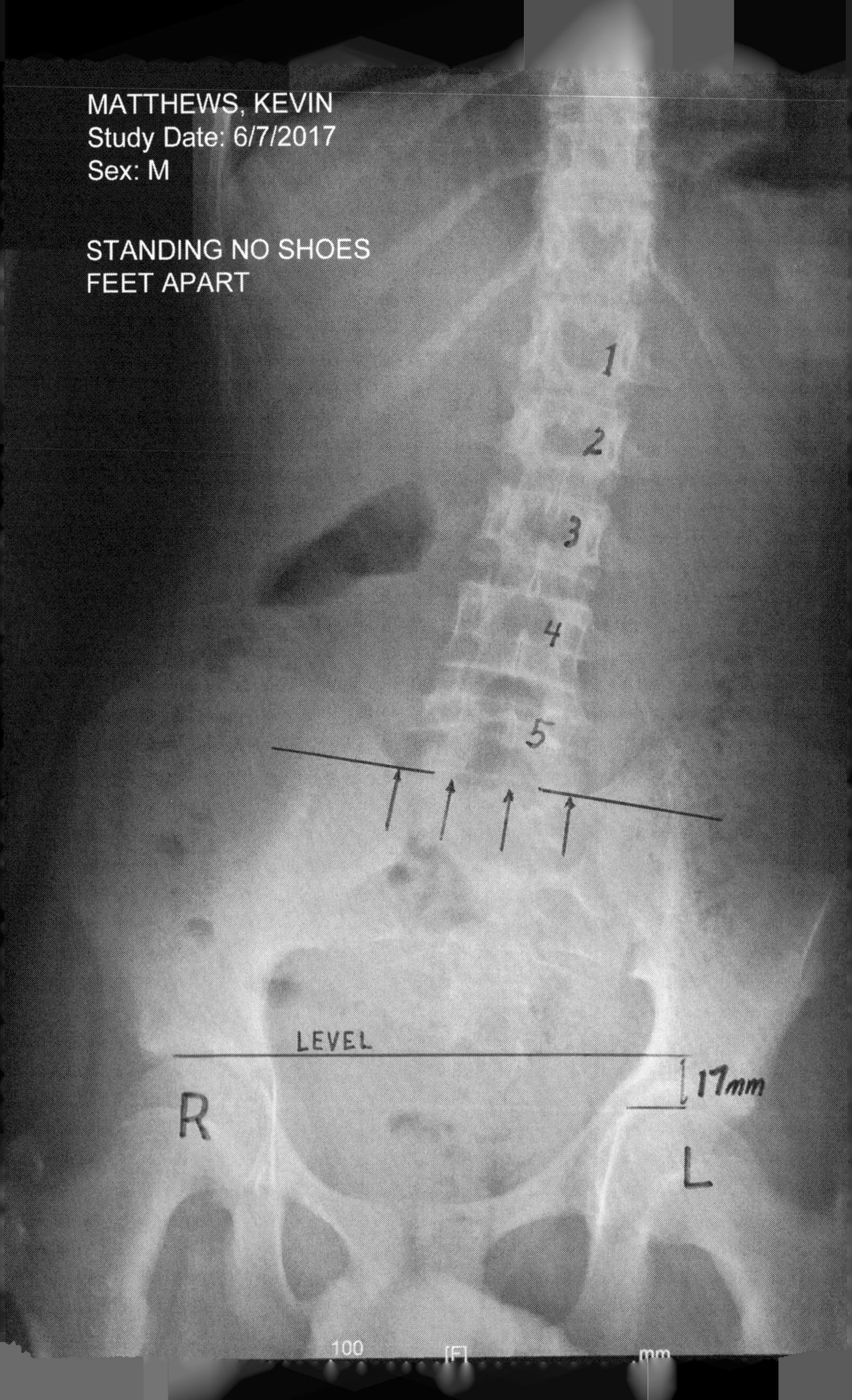

MATTHEWS, KEVIN
Study Date: 6/7/2017
Sex: M

STANDING NO SHOES
FEET APART

1
2
3
4
5

LEVEL
17mm

R
L

100 [F] mm

This is the x-ray previously mentioned of my patient Kevin Matthews, which clearly demonstrates a significant leg length difference of 17mm causing the top of the sacrum (see arrows) to be unlevel. Fortunately for Kevin, his scoliosis is functional at this point and simply the adapting curvature of a spine attempting to balance the torso atop an unlevel base. Note that the medical radiologist makes no mention of scoliosis or short leg and in fact misstates that the patient is leaning. Any pediatrician treating Kevin would have no idea that he has a short leg as they would typically see only the radiology report!

(Radiologists are not present during the taking of x-rays which are done by x-ray techs. Their comments about body postures are purely conjectural.) This lack of diagnostic information is a common oversight in the treatment of scoliosis.

NAME:SIGALOS,JANET
MRN: 065869
DOB: 4/18/1951, Sex: F
Acct #: 50172010121
ARRIVAL: 7/20/2017, D/C: 7/20/20

*** Final result ***

Ordering Provider:	Calvin Hargis, DC	*Authorizing Provider:*	Calvin Hargis, DC
Ordering Phone:	845-986-5500	*Authorizing Phone:*	
Ordering Fax:	845-986-6627	*Attending Provider:*	
Ordering Pager:		*PCP:*	

Other Ordering Provider:

Procedure:	**XR SPINE CERV PA LAT ODONT 3 V MAX [72040]**
Procedure Date:	07/20/2017 2:56 PM
Accession Number:	103514117
Order Number:	395895291
Ordering Diagnosis:	Subluxation complex of cervical region [M99.11 (ICD-10-CM)] Cervicalgia [M54.2 (ICD-10-CM)]
Reason for Exam:	pain
Performing Department:	DEPARTMENT
Patient Class:	OUTPATIENT

Study Result

Radiographs of the cervical spine

CLINICAL INFORMATION: Neck pain.

TECHNIQUE: Frontal and lateral views of the cervical spine were obtained. An odontoid view was obtained.

FINDINGS: Correlation is made with a prior study done on 08/05/2010.

The normal cervical lordosis is preserved. The cervical vertebral body height and alignment are maintained. The visualized pedicles appear intact. There is no evidence of acute bony fracture or destructive bony lesion.

Again noted is degenerative disc disease noted at the C5/6 level. The remaining cervical intervertebral disk spaces are preserved.

Again noted is posterior spurring noted at the C5/6 and C6/7 levels, more prominent at the C5/6 level.

There is no evidence of prevertebral soft tissue swelling noted.

IMPRESSION
IMPRESSION:

No evidence of acute bony fracture or subluxation.

Stable degenerative spondylosis of the lower cervical spine as described above. MR examination would be more sensitive for evaluation of disc pathology.

No significant change compared prior study done on 08/05/2010.

This radiographic report concerns my patient Janet Sigalos. Here the radiologist notes small bone spurs at C5-C6/C6-C7 and disc degeneration at C5 and C6 vertebrae. No mention is made of other pathology.

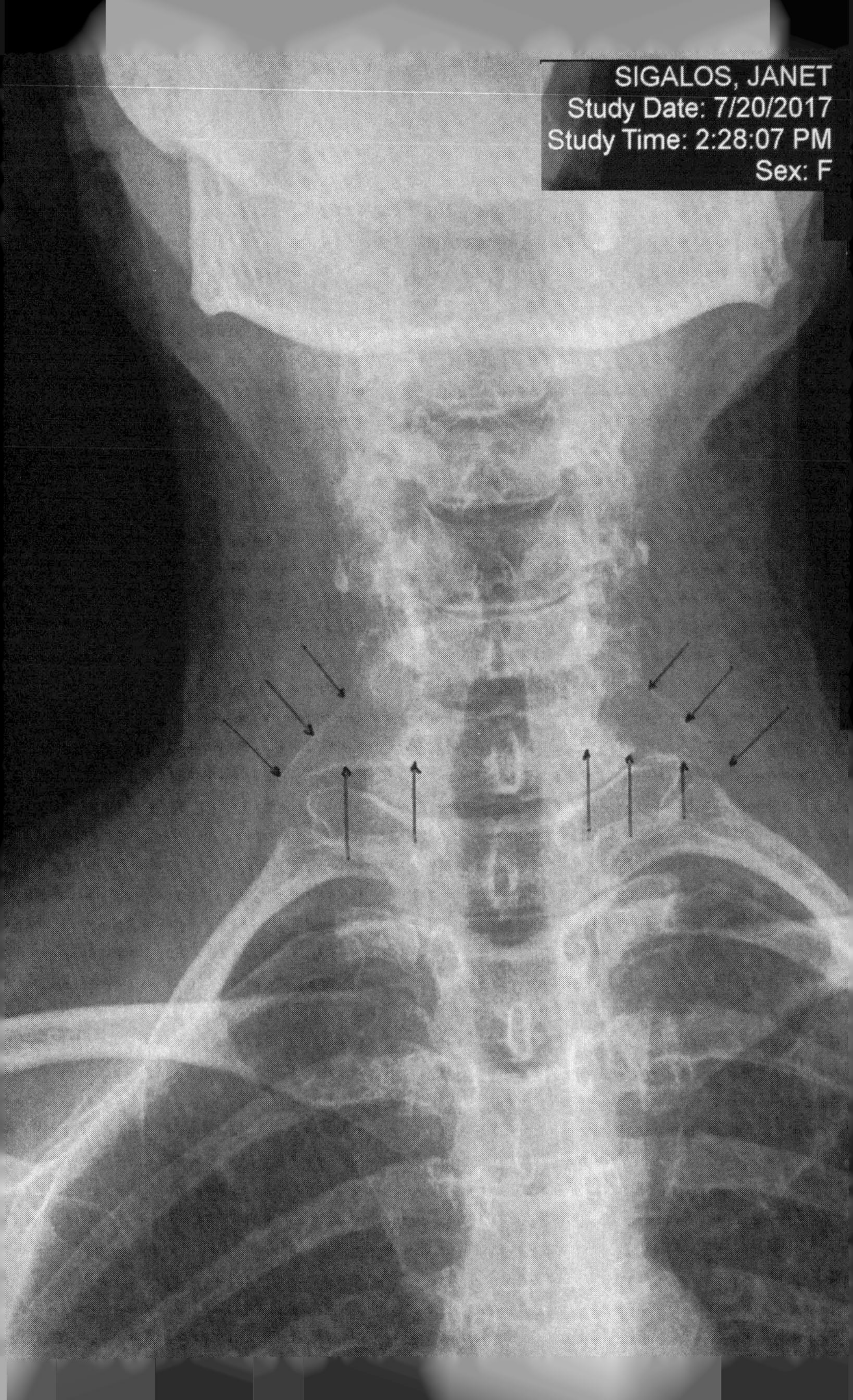
SIGALOS, JANET
Study Date: 7/20/2017
Study Time: 2:28:07 PM
Sex: F

Mrs. Sigalos has been plagued by shoulder and descending arm pain for months. The arrows reveal a large and abnormal outgrowth from the seventh cervical vertebrae known as a 'cervical rib', often responsible for compression and reduction of nerve and blood flow into the arms. No mention of this defect is made on the medical radiology report.

NAME:MUNLEY,RICHARD
MRN: 109030
DOB: 3/5/1955, Sex: M
Acct #: 50170030142
ARRIVAL: 1/3/2017, D/C: 1/3/2017

***** Final result *****

Ordering Provider:	Calvin Hargis, DC	*Authorizing Provider:*	Calvin Hargis, DC
Ordering Phone:	845-986-5500	*Authorizing Phone:*	
Ordering Fax:	845-986-6627	*Attending Provider:*	
Ordering Pager:		*PCP:*	None
Other Ordering Provider:			

Procedure: XR SPINE CERV 4 OR 5 V [72050]
Procedure Date: 01/03/2017 2:24 PM
Accession Number: 102766550
Order Number: 353979512

Ordering Diagnosis: Lumbalgia [M54.5 (ICD-10-CM)]
Cervicalgia [M54.2 (ICD-10-CM)]
Reason for Exam: Cervicalgia
Performing Department: [redacted] RADIOLOGY DEPARTMENT
Patient Class: OUTPATIENT

Study Result

Exam: Cervical spine, with oblique views.

Date and time:1/3/2017 2:10 PM

History: No reason given

Comparison: None

Findings:

There is normal curvature and alignment of the vertebral bodies. There is minimal osteophytes formation C5-C6 anteriorly. Intervertebral disc are unremarkable. Vertebral heights are maintained. Atlantoaxial relationships are preserved.

IMPRESSION
Impression:

Degenerative arthritis with minimal osteophytes formation C5-C6.
No fracture or dislocation.

THIS DOCUMENT HAS BEEN ELECTRONICALLY SIGNED BY [redacted] MD

Result History

XR SPINE CERV 4 OR 5 V (Order #353979512) on 1/3/2017 - Order Result History Report

This report of my patient Dr. Richard Munley mentions degeneration and minimal osteophytes (bone spurs) at the C5-C6 disc space only. The radiologist reports normal curvature and alignment of the cervical spine.

MUNLEY, RICHARD
ACC:102766550
Jan-03-2017
02:00:00 PM
Se: 1 (1)
m: 1/1

L
CW

ERECT

This is the x-ray mentioned in the preceding report. Dr. Munley had been experiencing a gradual loss of feeling and dexterity in his hands and feet for approximately two years. This lateral or side view x-ray of the cervical spine clearly indicates an abnormally straight cervical spine (vertical bar for comparison) and a backward slippage of the third cervical vertebrae C3 on the fourth cervical vertebrae C4. The medical radiologist's report states, "normal curvature and alignment of the vertebral bodies".

MUNLEY RICHARD
2017 Oct 05

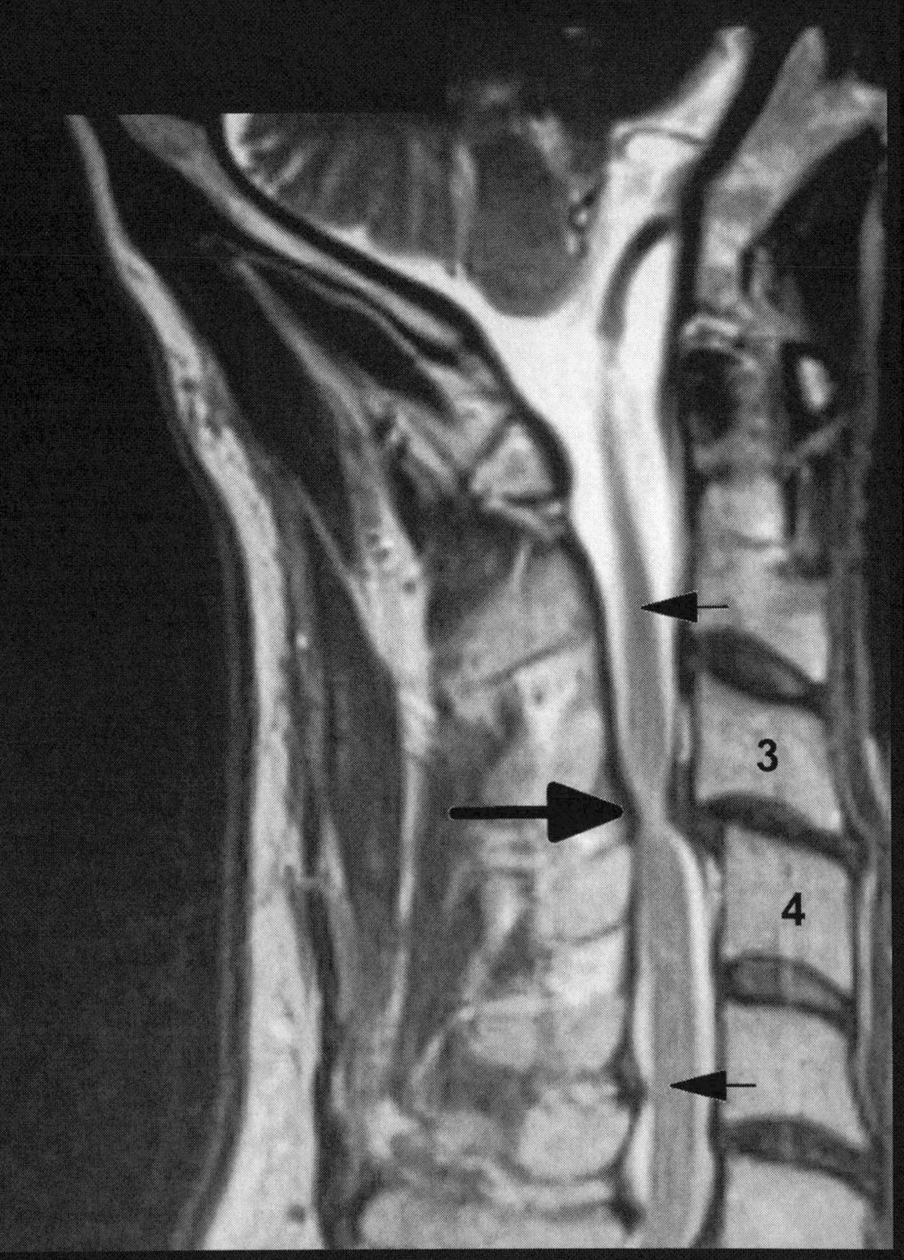

A follow-up MRI of Dr. Munley's cervical spine clearly depicts the backward slippage of C3 on C4. The spinal cord (gray vertical band marked by small arrows) demonstrates a profound indentation and spinal cord compression at C3-C4 consistent with his symptoms (large arrow). This is at a level of spinal cord injury that quadriplegics experience. In this case, the function of both the upper and lower extremities will become impaired over time and usually calls for surgical decompression to preserve function. (While chiropractic manipulation of C3 can reduce compressive symptoms, the chances of repositioning and stabilizing this major long-standing slippage is relatively low.) If the backward shift revealed on the previous x-ray had not been identified this MRI might never have been performed!

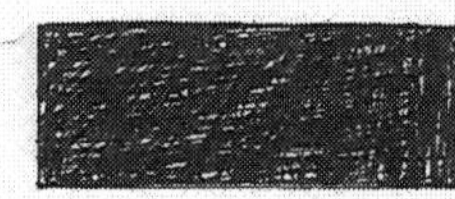

NAME:CROWDER,ANITA
MRN: 8031129
DOB: 2/7/1972, Sex: F
Acct #: 50180750056
ARRIVAL: 3/16/2018, D/C:

*** Final result ***

Ordering Provider:	Calvin Hargis, DC	*Authorizing Provider:*	Calvin Hargis, DC
Ordering Phone:	845-986-5500	*Authorizing Phone:*	845-986-5500
Ordering Fax:	845-986-6627	*Attending Provider:*	
Ordering Pager:		*PCP:*	
Other Ordering Provider:			

Procedure:	**XR SPINE CERV 4 OR 5 V [72050]**
Procedure Date:	03/16/2018 10:14 AM
Accession Number:	104435209
Order Number:	445219000
Ordering Diagnosis:	Vertebral subluxation complex of lumbar region [M99.13 (ICD-10-CM)] Lumbago [M54.5 (ICD-10-CM)] Subluxation complex of cervical region [M99.11 (ICD-10-CM)]
Reason for Exam:	Subluxation complex of cervical region, Cervicalgia
Performing Department:	HOSPITAL RADIOLOGY DEPARTMENT
Patient Class:	OUTPATIENT

Study Result

Radiographs of the cervical spine

performed on 3/16/2018 10:13 AM

for patient
female of 46 years

CLINICAL INFORMATION: Subluxation complex of cervical region, cervicalgia

TECHNIQUE: Frontal, oblique and lateral views of the cervical spine were obtained. An odontoid view was obtained.

FINDINGS: No previous examinations are available for review.

Cervical vertebral body heights are preserved. Cervical vertebral alignment is maintained. No fracture or destructive bone lesion is seen.

Cervical intervertebral disc spaces appear intact. Disc heights are maintained. No significant productive changes are found.

No neck soft tissue lesion is found.

IMPRESSION
IMPRESSION: Unremarkable radiographs of the cervical spine.

THIS DOCUMENT HAS BEEN ELECTRONICALLY SIGNED BY  MD

Anita Crowder was a young lady treated in my office. Due to her complaints of chronic neck and upper back pain and my examination, she was sent for spinal x-rays. Her x-ray report was provided by a medical radiologist. Their findings indicate a normal cervical spine stating, "Unremarkable radiographs of the cervical spine."

CROWDER, ANITA
Study Date: 3/16/2018

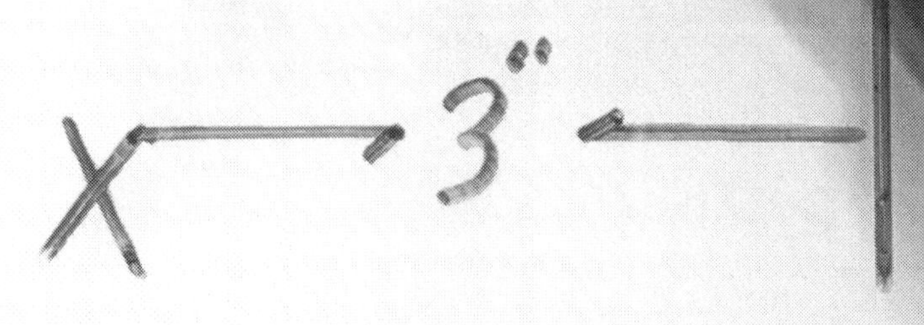

This is the lateral or side view x-ray of the cervical spine of Ms. Crowder mentioned in the report. The X in the radiograph rests at the center of her shoulder and like the vertical line and arrows mentioned below was placed there by myself upon examination of the x-ray films. The vertical line is drawn through the ear canal which represents the weight bearing center of the head and should be balanced directly over the X or mid-point of the shoulder. This radiograph reveals a severe forward head posture, FHP, and yet was read as a normal cervical spine x-ray by the medical radiologist! (Refer to FHP and the cascade of health effects evolving from this condition discussed earlier in this book.) Look closely at the small arrows and you will see the white, irregular, thickening of the joint surfaces reflecting arthritic changes at the junction of the lowest cervical vertebrae in the combined joints of the sixth, seventh and first thoracic vertebrae. Arthritis here is due to the excessive overloading of the lower spine by the forward head displacement.

Topics of Interest

Spinal Degeneration and Nerve Pain

Healthy spines have large nerve canals for the exiting nerve roots and can withstand bad posture and other forms of abuse. However, adults with degenerated spines (often found in seniors) have tight spinal canals that are significantly reduced and surrounded by degraded disc, bone, scar and joint tissue offering the nerve within no leeway or margin for compression.

Thus many older patients have flair-ups of joint or nerve (radicular) pain following relatively mild spinal stress when spinal joints swell further narrowing already compromised nerve canals. Due to the severity of pain and the ineffective treatment often received from health providers many of these patients seek chiropractic care within a few weeks of pain onset.

Unfortunately, many chiropractors hesitate to treat patients with severe spinal deterioration fearing worsening of their condition with manipulation. They should not, as close adherence to the protocols and therapy taught in this book can reduce joint swelling and nerve entrapment in a matter of days or weeks. In such situations, spinal manipulation can be avoided while proper therapy and home care effectively reduce the symptoms. Back sleeping with a single pillow under the neck and one under the legs should be strictly enforced. Those with neck pain should avoid crafting entailing neck flexion.

As in other cases mentioned in this book radicular pain may indicate a serious pathology and should be overseen by a competent health care provider.

Obesity and Low Back Pain

As was noted under the section on facet syndrome, excessive stomach fat increases lumbar lordosis and facet compression. Excess weight also places more load on the spinal joints, discs and joint cartilage of our hips, knees, ankles and feet. Moreover, many studies have shown that excess body weight increases inflammation throughout the body.[152] Obesity is a growing problem with 40% of adults and 20% of children overweight or obese.[153] The biggest culprits in the 'battle of the bulge' are fast foods, plate size, bad carbs (especially excess sugar) and no exercise. When my wife and I dine out we usually split the entree because most portions today are enormous making those who eat them enormous! You simply don't need that much. Learning to moderate will pay off handsomely.

Many carbohydrates like white bread, white rice, white potatoes, cookies, chips and sweets are quickly converted into glucose and then into fat leaving you hungry once again and unsatisfied. Following the glycemic index (GI) of carbohydrate foods can be helpful. The glycemic index rates foods numerically for how quickly they are converted to glucose in the body. Foods with numerical values over 55 are converted more quickly to glucose. Carbohydrates that break down slowly, releasing glucose gradually into the bloodstream, have a lower glycemic index, slower rates of digestion and offer a longer period before our hunger returns. A lower glycemic response equates to a lower insulin demand, better long-term blood glucose control and a reduction in blood lipids.

Recent animal research provides compelling evidence that high GI carbohydrates are associated with an increased risk of obesity. In one study, male rats were split in to high and low GI groups over 18 weeks. At studies end, the rats fed the high GI diet were 71%

fatter and had 8% less lean body mass than the low GI group.[154]

Losing weight is never easy and diets usually don't work because seldom do they teach proper eating habits. Consuming meals high in protein and veggies and low in bad carbs in sensible portions is essential. Combined with daily exercise for 30 minutes or more we can usually trim up to five pounds of weight per week in men and two to three pounds in women.

Starting your morning with a vegetable/fruit smoothie is a great way to begin to lose weight. An entire blender of veggies and some fruits are only about 300 calories. Adding a little juice, water or some other liquid of your choosing, makes two full glasses of delicious smoothie; enough for breakfast and lunch! Need more protein? Add a scoop of whey protein or a dollop of peanut butter and blend it up! (There are many recipes online.) You can save the other half for later; maybe breakfast tomorrow. A mixed legume salad with some chopped onion, pepper, carrot, celery or other vegetables with a little oil and vinegar, salt and pepper, makes for a tasty low calorie and very filling lunch that's easy to carry to work! Both are filled with fiber and antioxidants. A regular meal for dinner with sensible portions and low on cheap carbs is a nice ending meal for the day. You've eaten sensibly, gotten your exercise and hopefully won't be sitting with a bag of potato chips for the rest of the evening! Day one and done! Now do it for 30 more days and you won't believe the person your mirror will reveal at the end!

Anxiety and Pain

I don't think I can overstate the degree to which anxiety amplifies pain. I have literally taken histories from patients who were shaking in fear over their pain concerns. Will I have to live like this? Is it cancer? Am I going to lose my job because I can no longer do the work? How will I support my family? These are just a few of the questions that plague chronic pain sufferers as they traverse the pitfalls of chronic pain treatment in a world of practitioners ill-prepared to diagnose and treat chronic pain. As they dwell on these questions the impact of their pain becomes magnified by the endless loop of their self-doubts. Focus on their pain becomes a preoccupation that may consume the patient's waking hours, disrupting sleep and ramping up their anxiety to incredible heights. This hyper-vigilance has a profound effect on the brain causing pain centers to enlarge and become better 'wired' to magnify pain.[155,156,157]

Information and assurance by a knowledgeable health care provider can go a long way toward calming such fears. That's why after my history and clinical examination, I will review any imaging studies I have ordered on the following visit. This is done with the patient by my side, to educate them about the underlying sources of their pain. I can explain in simple terms, the reasons for their pain based on the pressures and forces being exerted on their spines and the soft tissue structures holding them together. Visualizing the spine in this manner also allows the chiropractor to construct a thoughtful plan for spinal manipulation, therapy and exercise rehab.

I have found no approach better able to calm patient fears than to render a clear and logical explanation of a patient's pain mechanism and then provide a treatment 'road map' back to health. An informed and educated patient, made aware of the mechanism of their pain and how we'll address it, is a patient now in control and with little need for anxiety. Unfortunately, finding a doctor able to dissect the underlying causes of musculoskeletal pain is uncommon for few have such intimate knowledge of spinal mechanics as the chiropractor.

Restful Sleep, Sleep Apnea and Obesity

Good and adequate sleep is important for healing and its loss has been heavily associated with fibromyalgia and persistent musculoskeletal complaints. Adequate rest is vital to healing! Unfortunately in our stressed and often overweight society the incidence of sleep apnea has grown exponentially with our hurried lifestyle and expanding waist size. Obstructive sleep apnea (OSA), is characterized by recurrent upper airway obstruction resulting in apneas (stopped breathing), hypopneas (shallow and incomplete breathing) and frequent sleep interruptions. Obstructive sleep apnea is closely linked by numerous studies to overweight and to a disorder termed Obesity Hypoventilation Syndrome (OHS). When we gain weight we also add fat to the soft tissues of our throats which can obstruct our breathing. This is magnified in sleeping positions and thus the dramatic rise in ventilation machines to assist breathing.

Continuous positive airway pressure (CPAP) therapy is a common treatment for obstructive sleep apnea. A CPAP machine uses a hose and mask or nose piece to deliver constant and steady air pressure. However these devices are often hard to get used to and come with a laundry list of possible problems: finding the proper size and fit, difficulty adjusting to the noise and pressure, maintaining a constant position in bed, difficulty tolerating forced air, chronic stuffy nose and dry mouth, claustrophobia, leaky mask and skin irritation including pressure sores, inability to fall asleep and chronic lung infections from poorly maintained or cleaned apparatus.

Surgical procedures such as midline partial glossectomy and or palatoplasty can be effective surgical modalities for the treatment of some pediatric and adult patients with mild to severe obstructive sleep apnea and involves surgical removal of tongue and palate tissue to open up one's airway. Statistics indicate that the majority of these surgeries result in good outcomes.

Losing weight can minimize and often eliminate the problem and the need for a respirator. According to the American College of Physicians, their first recommendation centers on weight loss for people who are overweight and obese. Losing just 10% of one's body weight can have a big effect on sleep apnea symptoms. In some cases, losing a significant amount of weight can even cure the condition.

Stomach Sleeping…A Good Way to Ruin Your Spine

Nobody sleeps on their stomach face down into our pillows. We turn either to the left or right. To compound the matter, most of those who stomach sleep use one or more pillows. Unfortunately, when we turn our necks to or near our maximum degree of rotation and then add an element of backward extension by virtue of our pillows, we stress the cervical spine constantly by stressing our delicate spinal joints and discs. This can accelerate spinal degeneration and be a leading factor in headache generation, neck and upper back pain, TMJ, balance issues and a host of other maladies also linked to brain stem and cervical nerve irritation. Stomach sleeping is one of the most stressing spinal postures and should be avoided for a healthy, disease-free cervical spine.

The Menacing Seat

We seldom think of a seat as being menacing but for many people with buttock, hip or upper leg pain this is an apt description. Man wasn't designed to sit for hours at a time but that's exactly what many of us do and today in their attempts to make seats 'ergonomic' or just plain cute designers have trended toward seats that curve up or in at their outside edges. As a result, many place undue pressure either at the hip or just behind the hip in the deep muscles of the upper leg and buttock. As we learned with micro-trauma this pressure might not be noticed on day one of getting a new car or desk chair but as the days pass and the hours of sitting add up the constant pressure from a raised or curved projection in our seat can begin to bruise and damage tissue.

It took me a while to understand this phenomenon and not until I had to solve my own hip and buttock pain, that I finally realized was being generated by an offending auto seat with an internal wire frame raised at the edges! This is a common pain generator and one generally overlooked. Fortunately, there is an easy fix. I advise patients to place a towel or other padding in the seat and to layer this in such a fashion as to level out the seat so that the edges can no longer 'jab' into those tender spots.

Cervical Pillows

Having treated thousands of patients for neck pain it's fairly common to hear of their bad experiences with cervical pillows! These are usually foam or some other form of contoured pillow specifically designed to curve into the neck. While it's true that for some small segment of these patients a curved pillow is helpful, for the vast majority they seem to cause more harm than good. The reason for this is pretty simple. Many neck pain sufferers begin using a new curved pillow to try to alleviate pain. The pain they experience however is often the result of a reversed, inflamed, strained or degenerated spine. As we have seen, areas of tissue inflammation, arthritic joints or degenerated discs do not like to be stressed. Few people have an optimal cervical curve to begin with and even fewer with the passage of time and aging. Therefore, the idea that one should sleep on a special curved or contoured pillow designed to hold the neck in a more perfect shape can be detrimental. Typically, a new neck complaint patient will give me their history and along the way tell me about the new neck pillow they've been using while their neck pain is getting worse. My advice is to skip the pillow unless specifically recommended by your chiropractor! Normally you should use a medium thickness pillow with a firm structure and in the manner discussed in this book.

Erect X-rays and MRI's for Spinal Complaints

When evaluating spinal pain erect 'weight bearing' x-rays and MRI's are needed for an accurate diagnostic. Taking either in an erect or sitting position places the spine under pressure during which abnormal postures and shifts of individual spinal vertebrae can be evaluated as can leg length differences and other sources of spinal or pelvic unleveling. Further, the true extent of spinal disc herniations can only be disclosed with weighted scans. In one study reported in the journal, World Neurosurgery in 2017, three hundred and ten patients with neck and arm pain underwent both a 'static' non-weighted MRI (lying down) and a 'dynamic' weighted MRI (sitting) of the cervical spine. The advantage of the weight-bearing MRI was that unlike an MRI lying down the sitting position allowed the patients to have additional studies done with the neck flexed and extended as well as in a neutral position. The static MRI demonstrated 156 disc herniations while the dynamic MRI revealed 186 disc herniations with related spinal cord compressions.[158] This should certainly be of interest to any patient suffering from spinal pain or any attorney representing an injury client!

Visit HealingTheHumanMachine.com for a video concerning weight-bearing x-ray and MRI.

Recumbent x-ray studies of the spine are largely inappropriate when one considers that most cases of spinal pain may involve mechanical abnormalities of the spine that are only manifest upon 'loading' of the neck or lower back upon standing. Standing or weight-bearing x-rays are therefore much more informative as to slippage and malposition of vertebrae and overloading of spinal structures in general and should be performed in all cases of chronic pain and acute neck, back, hip, pelvic or sciatic pain that hasn't improved following a week or two post-onset. Similarly, MRI studies are indicated in any prolonged cases of neck, back or other musculoskeletal pain that isn't resolving especially if they involve radiating pain into an extremity. Here again, weight-bearing MRI's will disclose much more spinal pathology than non-weight-bearing MRI's. Slippage of individual vertebra, abnormal compressions and many more and serious disc injuries will be disclosed when weight is placed upon the spine in weight-bearing images.

Book Bags and Kids

Spinal maturity occurs when the growth centers of spinal vertebrae are fully formed around age 18. Prior to this, the spine is softer and still in the process of converting to solid bone. Placing excessive loads on a developing and somewhat fragile young spine is risky as overloading can damage the developing growth centers in bone and result in distortions of adult bone shape! A child or young teen's book bag should be no more than 10 % of their weight. Some authorities suggest this can increase to 20% but I don't agree. I have taken many x-rays of farmworkers who began lifting at an early age only to note the irregular formation of spinal vertebrae as a result of overloading at an early age. The bottom line; weigh your child's backpack. If it's more than 10 percent of your child's weight contact their school and try to lighten their load!

Weather and Pain

Ever wonder why you hurt more with bad weather? Well the pressure of the mile of air above us exerts a fairly constant compressive force on each of us that we are hardly aware of. Every day, at sea level, we are exposed to an atmospheric pressure of approximately 14.7 pounds per square inch or one atmosphere of pressure on each part of our body. To illustrate this point, when we dive, water pressure at a depth of 9.8 m or 32 feet doubles this pressure. Bad weather conditions like rain or snow bring a 'low-pressure front' reducing the pressure of the air around us. A balloon at normal pressure will enlarge during rainy or snowy weather. So will your joints!

As joints swell, they stretch and activate pain-sensitive nerves increasing joint and muscular discomfort. This is one reason why even while following a correct regimen of therapy you may have a bad weather day or two in which pain seems to flare. If you should have more pain on a bad weather day don't be surprised!

Shaken Not Stirred

Major trauma, including serious car accidents and work injuries, may break bones but whether they do or not you can be sure soft tissue tearing will have occurred. Our bodies are held together by our soft tissues and violent accidents accelerate our body parts increasing G forces many times gravity tearing these tissues. Such trauma is unavoidable and often more severe than bone fractures. Broken bones mend, usually within six to eight weeks, but soft tissue injuries may last for months or years especially if treated inappropriately.

I remember the early seat belt commercials when an egg was placed in a model car without a restraint, rolled down a ramp and into a wall. The shell was broken on impact. However, it would have been far more accurate had the shell not been broken but the egg internally scrambled for the body's soft tissues can undergo tremendous damage largely unseen. As an authorized provider for workplace and auto injuries, I see many patients after having been treated by health providers who seem to have little understanding of soft tissue trauma. Still in pain, often worse than their original complaints, they usually relate overly aggressive prior care including stretch and massage, with no consideration of sleep postures or healing therapies.

This is truly unfortunate as in many states insurance regulations may allow for only a short window of treatment before an insurance company requires an 'independent review' of the injured party by an 'impartial' doctor. (Doctors who often make a lucrative income evaluating the degree of injury and the need for further care of accident victims; doctors, who in many cases would see far fewer insurance exams if they tended to be generous in their recommendations.) I know because I used to do insurance examinations. Most of these exams are handled through independent review companies employed by insurance carriers to 'distance' themselves from these reviews. Review companies often employ doctors who do multiple review exams per day. Many of these doctors, both medical and chiropractic, barely touch the patient, conducting brief and superficial exams and then issue cookie-cutter reports finding no further need for care. Following one examination in which I gave an opinion of more care needed and a causal relationship to a shoulder injury as a result of the accident, I was approached by the owner of the review company and ask to change my opinion. When I refused, no more reviews were sent my way. In many states, these exams may occur within as little as eight weeks post-injury! (Insurance companies lobby state and federal officials heavily (($$$$$)) to enact laws beneficial to their interests.)

Given the prevalence of improper treatment and the prolonged timeline of disc, joint, ligament, tendon and muscular healing, this trend toward quick and often biased examinations represents an egregious contempt for the injured. It would behoove lawmakers to carefully reconsider a more balanced shift toward empowering injury victims to have more time to treat and heal.

Tricks for Maintaining Healthy Sleep Positions

Our sleep positions are deeply ingrained into our psyche and hard to break. Invariably my patients start in the recommended sleep positions but shift while asleep. Over the years I've picked up a few tricks to ensure better compliance.

*To prevent stomach sleeping...sleep in a snug top and simply take a small float or 'fisherman's bobber' the size of an olive or somewhat larger, depress the button lifting the j hook, (normally used to attach the bobber to a fishing line), and attach the float to the garment just over the center of your breast bone (or in medical terms, the 'sternum').

*To prevent side sleep...try using pillows on either side of your body as you sleep supine. Alternately attaching small bobbers to a snug top along the lateral rib cage of the painful side often works. If all else fails sleep in a recliner.

*To prevent elevating a painful arm or shoulder over your head try tying a small cord loosely around the wrist of the painful extremity and attaching it to your lower sleep ware. A few inches of extra cord can ensure some movement but not enough to allow the arm to move above the shoulder area.

The Problem with NSAIDs

Non-steroidal anti-inflammatories are called NSAIDs. Many NSAIDs can be purchased without a prescription. Common types include; Aspirin (Bufferin, Bayer, and Excedrin), Ibuprofen (Advil, Motrin, Nuprin), Ketoprofen (Actron, Orudis) and Naproxen (Aleve).

NSAIDs work to block an enzyme called cyclo-oxygenase (COX) that is critical in your body's production of prostaglandins. Prostaglandins are made at sites of tissue damage or infection, where they cause inflammation, pain and fever as part of the healing process. When a blood vessel is injured, a prostaglandin called thromboxane stimulates the formation of a blood clot to try to heal the damage; it also causes the muscle in the blood vessel wall to contract, (causing the blood vessel to narrow), to try to prevent blood loss. Another prostaglandin called prostacyclin has the opposite effect to thromboxane, reducing blood clotting and removing any clots that are no longer needed; it also causes the muscle in the blood vessel wall to relax, so that the vessel dilates. The opposing effects that thromboxane and prostacyclin have on the width of blood vessels can control the amount of blood flow and regulate response to injury and inflammation. Taking NSAIDs may actually work against the healing process as the orderly healing of tissues is dictated largely by prostaglandins. Reducing them can reduce proper healing and lead to more scar and adhesive tissue and make for a more fragile and weakened repair more prone to re-injury! [159]

Prostaglandins produce the mucus coating that protects our stomach and gastrointestinal system from the acidic contents of the stomach. These stomach acids break down our food and without prostaglandins to provide this mucus barrier, the stomach acids can produce ulcerations of the esophagus, stomach or intestines. NSAIDs cause high rates of gastrointestinal problems causing ulcers and other problems in your esophagus, stomach, or small intestine as they inhibit prostaglandin production.[160]

In 2017 the FDA (Food and Drug Administration) strengthened its warning concerning NSAIDs other than aspirin, stating that there is now increased concern that they can provoke heart attack and stroke leading to death as early as in the first few weeks of taking these medications.

NSAIDs have also been linked to miscarriage especially in the early months of pregnancy, which has again necessitated a further warning from the FDA.[161,162] Acetominophen, (not considered an NSAID due to its low anti-inflammatory properties), has also been linked to the increased risk of attention deficit hyperactivity disorder (ADHD) in children born to mothers who took this medication at any time during pregnancy!

Furthermore, NSAIDs reduce the blood flow to the kidneys, which makes them work more slowly. Reduced blood flow can eventually lead to kidney failure and require dialysis. When your kidneys are not working well, fluid builds up in your body resulting in higher blood pressure. If your arteries are already compromised because you are a smoker or have arterial restriction due to atherosclerotic plaque, damage may occur to organs like the brain or placenta by altering arterial blood supply to these and other organs.

NSAIDs can also cause extreme allergic reactions, especially in people with asthma. Experts aren't sure why. Many specialists recommend that people who have asthma avoid them. Prostaglandins are also important in regulating the contraction and relaxation of the muscles of the gut during digestion, our airways in respiration and in regulating the female reproductive system and ovulation.

Natural Anti-Inflammatory Aids for Healing

For several years now my primary recommendation for an anti-inflammatory has been curcumin. Curcumin is the active ingredient in turmeric that gives it much of its anti-inflammatory properties. Curcumin has some interesting effects on the body. Research studies indicate that this amazing compound has the potential to lessen, prevent or even cure a wide range of health conditions like heart disease, bronchitis and asthma, depression, fatigue, Alzheimer's disease, rheumatoid arthritis and osteoarthritis, cancer, irritable bowel syndrome, leukemia, cirrhosis, psoriasis and speeds wound healing. The percentage of curcumin in turmeric is low however, only 2% to 5% of its dry weight.

I recommend that my patients take 95% pure curcumin which has been extracted from turmeric. Pure curcumin is available through various companies online. Normally I recommend patients take a level teaspoon once per day or up to three 1000 milligram capsules, one with each meal. Mixing curcumin with modest amounts of black pepper greatly increases its absorption by as much as 2000%. Piperine, an alkaloid found in black pepper, is responsible. Curcumin is also fat-soluble. Without fat, the compound doesn't dissolve properly and then curcumin has difficulty being absorbed through the gut and into the bloodstream; healthy fats like avocado, olive and coconut oil increases absorption as well. Finally, quercetin, a plant flavonoid found in red wine and many fruits and vegetables, blocks enzymes that reduce curcumin.

A small smoothie with fruit, greens and veggies, along with curcumin and a little black pepper morning and evening can be very effective in fighting inflammation and are loaded with vitamins and minerals. An anti-inflammatory method of eating known as the Mediterranean diet, is a healthy style of eating and could include; tomatoes, beets, olive oil, coconut oil, flax oil, green leafy vegetables such as spinach, kale, collards, celery, Bok Choy, Swiss chard, nuts like almonds and walnuts, chia and flax seeds, fatty fish like salmon, mackerel, tuna, and sardines, fruits such as strawberries, blueberries, cherries, apples, pineapple and oranges and spices like cinnamon, ginger and turmeric .

Curcumin is a blood thinner and should not be taken with medications to reduce blood clotting nor by diabetics as it may lower blood sugar. Although uncommon, other side effects may occur with certain medications and I advise you consult your pharmacist if on medication before taking curcumin. One should research the benefits and risks of taking this or any other neutraceutical or medication before beginning.

Falling in the Elderly

Falls are the leading cause of fatal injury and the most common cause of nonfatal hospital admissions among older adults. Good balance is maintained as sensors in the cervical spine report information on balance to the brain and inner ear.

But when misalignment and degeneration of the cervical spine degrade and interrupt this messaging good balance is diminished. In an interesting study, sixty-seven patients with staggering and balance issues were evaluated before and just after having cervical spine manipulations. These patients demonstrated marked improvement in balance after their adjustment.[144] These findings have been reduplicated many times including one study by Galm and colleagues who saw a 77.4% reduction in vertigo and dizziness in 31 seniors receiving cervical spine manipulation.[70,163]

Spinal manipulation must be combined with leg strengthening exercises in the elderly, who quickly lose leg strength without an active exercise regimen. This can be accomplished easily with dining room chairs. I have my senior patients place two chairs with their backs facing and body width apart. Stepping between, I ask them to hold on to the backs of the chairs as I have them do a gentle squat and then as they rise, to do a toe lift. Starting slowly with just a few repetitions and with supervision in the beginning, seniors can easily ramp up leg strength within a few weeks by adding a few more squats and lifts as they become stronger.

Visit HealingTheHumanMachine.com for a video demonstrating these exercises.

Baby Needs an Adjustment Too

Babies have spines and being born can be traumatic. Passing through the birth canal places tremendous pressure on the newborn; forces easily capable of shifting spinal vertebrae. Learning to walk can also be punishing. The falls and minor mishaps that children endure can damage and subluxate the spine. As a result of these stresses and injuries, the tiny spinal vertebrae of newborns and young children may become misaligned resulting in localized pain, inflammation and irritation of target organs supplied by the spinal nerves emanating from affected vertebrae.

In chronic ear infections misalignment of the topmost spinal vertebrae (the atlas), situated just below the skull and sitting in close approximation to the inner ear, can create localized pressure and irritation when it shifts laterally out of position toward the affected ear. This was the case with my second grandchild who was faced with the prospect of having tubes inserted surgically into the ear when her chronic ear infections got out of hand. Living some hours away I recommended she be seen by a chiropractor in her town who rendered eight to ten gentle spinal adjustments to reposition her wayward atlas. This therapy rendered over six weeks left two-year-old Katie with a complete and lasting resolution of her ear complaints.

Especially common are babies born with 'wry neck' or torticollis and colic. Each condition may be related to the misalignment of the spine. The onset of torticollis or 'wry' neck is easy to understand as the battering of the head through the birth canal can damage and misalign the cervical vertebrae and be greatly improved with gentle adjustments. Throughout my practice I have had the pleasure of providing relief for this condition as well as colic when a misalignment of vertebrae in the mid-back has resulted in localized pain or stomach upset.

Asthma is amenable to chiropractic manipulation of the spine as well. Adjustments of the mid and upper back have diminished asthma symptoms for many but not all of my younger patients. An interesting study was conducted by Bronfort and colleagues. 36 patients aged 6 to 17 years with mild and moderate persistent asthma were admitted to a study in which approximately half received twenty chiropractic spinal adjustments over a three-month period. Asthma severity ratings showed a reduction of 39% and the overall improvement rating was 50% to 75%. The changes in patient-rated severity and the improvement rating remained unchanged at a 12-month post-treatment follow-up.[164]

It should be understood that although spinal misalignment may be related to almost any health condition this is just one of many possible causations. Having said this however, it is my strong belief that the spine should be considered a factor in most disease processes and given a proper evaluation.

Growing Pains

During my many years in practice, I have encountered numerous children whose pediatrician has dismissed their complaints of headaches, foot, leg, hip, spinal or other forms of pain as 'growing pains'. Growing should never be painful and when it is, your child's body is sending a message that something is wrong. Childhood complaints might follow from something as benign as a mild muscle strain, bump or bruise and if so be of short duration and usually of little concern. However, complaints that are voiced over a longer time frame should never be dismissed, as childhood development is a slow and evolving process that can easily go wrong. Children are subject to many of the same maladies as adults. These include abnormalities of spinal or other structural development such as scoliosis, leg length difference, postural abnormalities of the legs, ankles and feet, forward carriage of the head, reversed curvature of the cervical spine and a host of other conditions. Never discount your child's complaints and also remember children who have pain from an early age may accept their discomfort as normal. When in doubt see a competent musculoskeletal expert.

Growing should never be painful and when it is, your child's body is sending a message that something is wrong. One of the biggest mistakes that parents make is never taking a good and thoughtful look at their child's body conformation.

The Managed Care Scam

While actors and ex-athletes are employed to convince you of the benefits of low-cost or no-cost managed health care, beware. They don't call these plans managed for no reason. In fact, they often manage you right out of the benefits they promise! Imagine you need a needed test or have been advised on a course of treatment only to find that a 'case manager' for your insurance company, whom you've never seen, has deemed the test or treatment unnecessary. Or, having been placed in a hospital with orders for a multi-day course of treatment to be told your care is being reviewed by your insurance provider, then handed a bill whopping for out-of-pocket expenses due to insurance non-approval or their low reimbursement levels. Insurance is a numbers game; if they pay out more than they take in they lose. Insurance companies do not like to lose. They like to profit. And it is insurance greed that is dramatically reducing the quality of health care in America.

As a health provider, it is common to have patients pay a $40 co-pay while I receive a check from the insurance company for $1.19. And yet they call the shots. After paying huge premiums you can't afford to go to a doctor not enrolled in your plan. At the same time, doctors are dropping these plans due to onerous and redundant paperwork often processed by poorly trained staff routed through call centers in India or other locations when knowledge of your plan and language is often a barrier. This includes many Medicare Advantage plans where believe me the insurance company has the advantage! My advice, especially for seniors is to stick to regular Medicare and secondary insurance endorsed by AARP, (the American Association of Retired Persons).

The Doctor Has a Problem

While in graduate school, I was sitting one morning with my two-year-old son on my lap. As I was lifting and twisting to place him on the floor, I felt a strong stab of pain in my mid-back which left me unable to take a deep breath! I literally could not take a full breath as each time I attempted to do so, my efforts were meant with stabbing mid-back and radiating rib pain. Early in my chiropractic training, I realized that the twisting and bending movement had displaced one of my thoracic vertebra and the rib head with which it joined! (The ribs insert into and form joints with the vertebrae of the thoracic spine. Sudden displacement or 'subluxation' of this kind, leaves you laboring for a complete breath you cannot achieve and in severe pain. This is one of the rare exceptions when the surrounding muscle structures do go into spasm including the muscles between and adjacent to the affected ribs.) I remained in agony for the next several hours until a senior student adjusted and reseated my spine and rib head into position. Spinal manipulation brought me instant relief. Although uncommon, rib head displacement is a painful ordeal.

Look at Yourself or Those You Care About

I have a habit of constantly evaluating the posture of those around me. I can hardly walk down a street without noting the people limping with a bad hip or knee, often due to their leg length difference, so obvious to me but unknown to them. Or the 'humped' and rounded backs of those who chronically side sleep. Those with worn-out 'knock knees' and severe bunions due to their flat feet and ankle pronation. Young adults and teens with forward head displacement from texting and computer overuse. It is rare however, to find a patient aware of their own body deformities. Now as you come to the end of this book, I hope you will have acquired a keener eye for your body imbalances and those of the people you care about. Good biomechanical balance and movement is the key to healthy, pain-free longevity.

Final Words

I would like to thank the many fine doctors of Palmer Chiropractic College and New York Chiropractic College, for their wisdom and love for this profession which they imparted to me and to the thousands of my patients who continued my education. I hope this book provides illumination to dispel some of the confusion that has surrounded the treatment of musculoskeletal conditions and will serve as a basis for better collaboration between health care providers of every sort recognizing what each profession can offer for the benefit of their patients.

1. Von Korff, M., Deyo, R., Cherkin, D., Barlow, W. Back pain in primary care. Outcomes at 1 year. Spine (Phila Pa 1976). 1993 Jun 1;18(7):855-862.

2. Hansson, T., Hansson, E. The effects of common medical interventions on pain, back function, and work resumption in patients with chronic low back pain: A prospective 2-year cohort study in six countries. Spine (Phila Pa 1976). 2000 Dec 1;25(23):3055-3064.

3. The PainSTORY survey was conducted by an independent research company, Ipsos MORI, in collaboration with the following independent third parties: *f* European Federation of IASP Chapters *f* World Institute of Pain *f* OPEN Minds.

4. Croft, P., Macfarlane, G., Papageorgiou, A., Thomas, E., Silman, A. Outcome of low back pain in general practice: a prospective study. BMJ 1998;316:1356-1359 (2 May).

5. Prescription Drug Use And Persons Age 45+, AARP, June 2002.

6. Kolodny, A., Courtwright, D., Hwang, C., Kreiner, P., Eadie, J., Clark, T., Alexander, G. The prescription opiod and heroin crisis: public health approach to an epidemic of addiction. Anu Rev Public Health. 2015;36:1-25.

7. Van Zee, A. The promotion and marketing of OxyContin: commercial triump, public tragedy. Am J Public Health. 2009;99:221-227.

8. Chen, J., Humphreys, K., Shah, N. Lembke, A. Distribution of opioids by different types of Medicare prescribers. JAMA Intern Med. 2015;176:259-261

9. Volkow, N., McLellan, T., Cotto, J., Karithanom, M., Weiss, S. Characteristics of opioid prescriptions in 2009. JAMA. 2011; 305: 1299-1301.

10. Levy, B., Paulozzi, L,, Mack, K., Jones, C. Trends in opioid analgesic-prescribing rates by specialty, U.S., 2007-2012. Am J Prev Med. 2015:1-5.

11. Soteri, P., Gunderson, E., Levin, F., Training Physicians To Treat Substance Use Disorders. Curr Psychiatry Rep. 2008 Oct; 10(5): 399–404.

12. Karon, A. Medical schools respond to the opioid epidemic. Medical Education 2017.

13. Day, C., Yeh, A., Franko, O., Ramirez, M., Krupat, E. Musculoskeletal medicine: an assessment of the attitudes and knowledge of medical students at Harvard Medical School. Acad Med. 2007 May; 82(5):452-457.

14. DiGiovanni, B., Sundem, L., Southgate, R., Lambert, D. Musculoskeletal Medicine Is Underrepresented in the American Medical School Curriculum. Clin Orthop Relat Res. 2016 Apr;474(4):901-7

15. Deyo, R., Mirza, S., Martin, B. Back pain prevalence and visit rates: estimates from U.S. national surveys, 2002. Spine. 2006;31:2724-7.

16. Friedly, J., Chan, L., Deyo, R. Increases in lumbosacral injections in the Medicare population:1994-2001. Spine. 2007;32:1754–60.

17. Deyo, R., Gray, D., Kreuter, W., Mirza, S., Martin, B. United States trends in lumbar fusion surgery for degenerative conditions. Spine. 2005;30:1441–5.

18. Martin, B., Mirza, S., Comstock, B., Gray, D., Kreuter, W., Deyo, R. Are lumbar spine reoperation rates falling with greater use of fusion surgery and new surgical technology? Spine. 2007;32:2119–26.

19. Paulozzi, L., Budnitz, D., Xi, Y. Increasing deaths from opioid analgesics in the United States. Pharmacoepidemiol Drug Saf. 2006;15:618–27.

20. Meier, B. 3 officials are sentenced in case involving OxyContin. The New York Times; Jul 21, 2007. p. C4.

21. Abelson, R. Medtronic will settle accusations on kickbacks. The New York Times; Jul 19, 2006. p. C4.

22. Abelson, R. Financial ties are cited as issue in spine study. The New York Times; Jan 30, 2008.

23. Mitchell, J. Utilization trends for advanced imaging procedures: evidence from individuals with private insurance coverage in California. Medical Care. 2008;46:460–6.

24. Weiner, D., Kim, Y., Bonino, P., Wang, T. Low back pain in older adults: are we utilizing healthcare resources wisely? Pain Med. 2006;7:143–50.

25. Lurie, J., Birkmeyer, N., Weinstein, J. Rates of advanced spinal imaging and spine surgery. Spine. 2003:28:616-20

26. Swedlow, A., Johnson, G., Smithline, N., Milstein, A. Increased costs and rates of use in the California workers' compensation system as a result of self-referral by physicians. N Engl J Med. 1992;327(21):1502–1506.

27. Mitchel, J. Do financial incentives linked to ownership of specialty hospitals affect physicians' practice patterns? Medical Care. 2008;46:732-7.

28. Rao, J., Kroenke, K., Mihaliak, K., Eckert, G. Weinberger M. Can guidelines impact the ordering of magnetic resonance imaging studies by primary care providers for low back pain? Am J Manag Care. 2002 Jan; 8(1):27-35

29. Mirza, S., Deyo, R., Heagerty, P., Turner, J., Martin, B., Comstock, B. One-year outcomes of surgical versus nonsurgical treatments for discogenic back pain: a community-based prospective cohort study. Department of Orthopaedic Surgery and The Dartmouth Institute for Health Policy and Clinical Practice, Geisel School of Medicine at Dartmouth, Hanover, NH

30. Nguyen, T., Randolph, D., Talmage, J., Sussop, P., Travis, R. Long-term outcomes of lumbar fusion among workers' compensation subjects: a historical cohort study. Spine 2011 Feb 15;36(4):320-31.

31. Arts, M., Kols, N., Onderwater, S., Peul, W. Clinical Outcomes of Instrumental Fusion for the Treatment of Failed Back Surgery Syndrome: a Case Series of 100 Patients. Acta Neurochirurgica (wen), 2012 July:154(7): 1213-1217

32. Deyo, R., Hallvik, S., Hildebran, C., Marino, M., O'Kane, N., Carson, J., Van Otterloo, J., Wright, D., Millet, L., Wakeland, W. Use of prescription opioids before and after an operation for chronic pain (lumbar fusion surgery)PAIN: March 06. 2018.

33. Ebenbichler, G., Leitgeb, J., Amtmann, G., Konig, F., Schernthaner, M., Resch K., Kainberger, F. Degeneration and Instability and the Relation to Patients' Function Late After Lumbar Disc Surgery: Data from a 12-Year Follow-Up. Am J Phys Med Rehabil. 2016 Dec;95(12):871-879.

34. Bigos, S, Bowyer, O., Braen, G., et al. Acute Low Back Problems in Adults. Clinical Practice Guideline, Quick Reference Guide Number. 14. Rockville, MD: U.S. Department of Health and Human Services, Public Health Service, Agency for Health Care Policy and Research, AHCPR Pub. No. 95-0643. December 1994.

35. Haldeman, S. Sudden Neck Movement and Cervical Artery Dissection: The Chiropractic Experience. CMAJ 2001; 165 (7): 905–906,

36. Cassidy, J., Boyle, E., Cote, P., He, Y., Hogg-Johnson, S., Silver, F., Bondy, S. Risk of vertebrobasilar stoke and chiropractic care: results of a population-based case-control and case-crossover study. Spine (Phila Pa 1976). 2010 Mar 1;35(5):595

37. Lucian, L. Incidence of Adverse Events and Negligence in Hospitalized Patients Results of the Harvard Medical Practice Study. Ne w England Journal of Medicine 1991 (Feb 7): 324 (6): 370-376

38. Null, G., Dean, C., Feldman, M., Rasio, D., Smith, D. March 2004, Life Extension Magazine "Death by Medicine"

39. Nyiendo, J., Haas, M., Goodwin, P. Patient characteristics, practice activities, and one-month outcomes for chronic, recurrent low-back pain treated by chiropractors and family medicine physicians: a practice-based feasibility study. Journal of Manipulative and Physiological Therapeutics 2000 May;23(4):239-45

40. Croft, P., Macfarlane, G., Papageorgiou, A., Thomas, E., Silman, A. Outcome of low back pain in general practice: a prospective study. BMJ 1998;316:1356-1359

41. Smucker, D., Konrad, T., Curtis, P., Carey, T. Practitioner Self-confidence and Patient Outcomes in Acute Low Back Pain, Arch Fam Med. 1998;7:223-228.

42. Kazis, et al. (2019), BMJ Open

43. Goertz, et al. (2013), Spine

44. Korthals-de Bos, et al. (2003), British Medical Journal

45. Nyiendo, et al. (2000), Journal of Manipulative and Physiological Therapeutics

46. Goertz, et al. (2018) JAMA Open Network

47. Schneider, et al. (2015), Spine

48. Keeney, et al. (2012), Spine

49. Haas, et al. (2005), Journal of Manipulative and Physiological Therapeutics

50. Hoving, et al. (2002), Annals of Internal Medicine

51. McCrory, Penzlen, Hasselblad, Gray. (2001), Duke Evidence Report

52. Boline, et al. (1995), Journal of Manipulative and Physiological Therapeutics

53. Bronfort, et al. (2012), Annals of Internal Medicine

54. Hurwitz, et al. (2016), Journal of Manipulative and Physiological Therapeutics

55. Weeks, et al. (2016), Journal of Manipulative and Physiological Therapeutics

56. Liliedahl, et al. (2010), Journal of Manipulative and Physiological Therapeutics

57. Adams, et al. (2017) Spine

58. Hertzman-Miller, et al. (2002), American Journal of Public Health

59. Meeker, Haldeman. (2002), Annals of Internal Medicine

60. Grunhagen, T., Wilde, G., Soukane, D., Shirazi-Adl, S., Urban J. Nutrient supply and intervertebral disc metabolism. J Bone Joint Surg Am. 2006 Apr;88 Suppl 2:30-5.

61. Thiry, P., Reumont, F., Brismee, J., Dierick, F. Short-term increase in discs' apparent diffusion is associated with pain and mobility improvements after spinal mobilization for low back pain. SciRep. 2018 May 29;8(1):8281. doi: 10.1038/s41598-018- 26697 -7.

62. Cramer, G., Fournier, J.,Wolcott, C., Henderson, C. Degenerative Changes Following Spinal Fixation in a Small Animal Model, J Manipulative Physiol Ther 2004 (Mar): 27 (3): 141-154

63. Morgan, D., Proske, U. Popping Sarcomere Hypothesis Explains Stretch Induced Muscle Danage. Proceedings of the Australian Pharmacological Society (2004) 34: 19-23

64. Huard, J., Li, Y., Fu, F. Muscle Injuries and Repair. Current Trends in Research. Journal of American Bone and Joint Surgery. 84(5):822-832, 2002

65. Tidus, P., Shoemaker, J. Effleurage massage, muscle blood flow and long-term post-exercise strength recovery. Int J Sports Med 1995 Oct;16(7):478-83

66. Tidus, P. Manual Massage and recovery of muscle function following exercise: a literature review. J Orthop Sports Phys Ther 11997 Feb;25(2):107-12

67. Kames, J., Burton, H. Continuous therapeutic ultrasound accelerates repair of contraction-induced skeletal muscle damage in rats. Arch Phys Med Rehabil 2002 Jan;83(1):1-4

68. Bogduk, N., Govind, J. Cervicogenic headache: an assessment of the evidence on clinical diagnosis, invasive tests, and treatment. Lancet Neurol 2009; 8:959.

69. Raczkowski, J., Daniszewska, B., Zolynski, K. Functional scoliosis caused by leg length discrepancy. Archives of Medical Science 2010 Jun 30; 6(3):393-398

70. Humphreys, K., Peterson, C. Comparison of outcomes in neck pain patients with and without dizziness undergoing chiropractic treatment: a prospective cohort study with 6 month follow-up. Chiropractic & Manual Therapies 2013 (Jan &): 21:3

71. Brennan, T., Leape, L., Laird, N,.Hebert, L., Localio, A., Lawthers, A., Newhouse, J., Weiler, P., Hiatt, H. Results of the Harvard Medical Practice Study I. Incidence of Adverse Events and Negligence in Hospitalized Patients. New England Journal of Medicine 1991 (Feb7): 324(6): 370-376

72. Lee, W., Okeson, J., Lindroth, J. The Relationship Between Forward Head Posture and Temporomandibular Disorders, J Orofac Pain 1995 (Spr): 9(2): 161-167

73. Watson, D., Trott, P. Cervical Headache: An Investigation of Natural Head Posture and Upper Cervical Flexor Muscle Performance. Cephalalgia 1993 (Aug); 13 (4): 272–284

74. Kapandji, A. The Physiology of the Joints:The Trunk and the Vertebral Column, Volumn 3

75. Cailliet, R., Gross, L. Rejuvenation Strategy. New York, Doubleday and Co. 1987

76. Sperry, R. (1988) Roger Sperry's Brain Research. Bulletin of The Theosophy Science Study Group 26 (3-4), 27-28

77. Cobzeanu, M., et al. The implications of cervical spine degenerative and traumatic diseases in the pathogenesis of cervical vertigo and hearing loss. Rev Med Chir Soc Med Nat Iasi. 2009 Jul-Sep;113(3):814-8

78. Netter, F. High Cervical Spine: C1–C2. Atlas of Human Anatomy

79. Purves, D. (2011). Neuroscience (5. ed.). Sunderland, Mass.: Sinauer. p. 740. ISBN 978-0-87893-695-3

80. Hoffman, D. Treatment of carpal tunnel syndrome: is there a role for local corticosteroid injection? Neurology 2006;66(3):459-460.

81. Hui, A., Wong, S., Leung, C., Tong, P., Mok, V., Poon, D., Li-Tsang, C., Wong, L., Boet, R. A Randomized controlled trial of surgery vs. steroid injection for carpal tunnel syndrome. Neurology. 2005;64(12): 2074-2078.

82. Atroshe, I., Gummesson, C., Ornstein, E., et al. Carpal tunnel syndrome and keyboard use at work: a population-based study. Arthritis Rheum. 2007;56(11):3620-3625.

83. Piazzini, D., Aprilr, I., Ferrara, P., et al. A systematic review of conservative treatment of carpal tunnel syndrome. Clin Rehabil. 2007;21(4):299-314.

84. Gionis, T., Groteke, E. Surgical Alternatives: Spinal Decompression. Orthopedic Technology Review, 2003; 6(5).

85. Gundersen, B., Henrie, M., Cristensen, J. A Clinical Trial on Non-Surgical Spinal Decompression Using vertebral Axial Distraction Delivered by a Computerized Traction Device. The Academy of Chiropractic Orthopedists, Quarterly Journal of ACO, June 2004.

86. Shealy, N., Borgmeyer, V. Decompression, Reduction, and Stabilization of the Lumbar Spine: A Cost-Effective Treatment for Lumbosacral Pain. American Journal of Pain Management Vol. 7 No. 2 April 1997.

87. Kraemer, J., Kolditz, D., Gowin, R. Water and eletrolyte content of human intervertebral discs under variable load. Spine 1985 Jan-Feb; 10(1):69-71.

88. Adams, M., Hutton, W. The effect of posture on the role of the apophyseal joints in resisting intervertebral compressive forces. J Bone Surg (UK) 1980;62(3):358-362.

89. Raczkowski, J., Daniszewska, B., Zolynski, K. Functional scoliosis caused by leg-length discrepancy. Arch Med Sci. 2010;6(3):393-398.

90. Knutson, G. Anatomic and functional leg-length inequality: a review and recommendation for clinical decision-making. Part 1, anatomic leg-length inequality: prevalence, magnitude, effects and clinical significance. Chiropr Osreopat. 2005;13:11.

91. Golightly, Y., Allen, K., Helmick, C., Renner, J., Jordan, J. Symptoms of the knee and hip in individuals with and without limb length inequality. Osteoarthr Cartilage. 2009;17(5):596-600.

92. Henchoz, Y., de Goumoens, P., Norberg, M., Paillex, R., So, K. Role of physical exercise in low back pain rehabilitation: a randomized controlled trial of a three-month exercise program in patients who have completed multidisciplinary rehabilitation. Spine. 2010;35(12):1192-1199.

93. Cummings, G., Scholz, J., Barnes, K. The effect of imposed leg length difference on pelvic bone symmetry. Spine. 1193;18(3):368-373.

94. Norkin, C., Levangie, P. Joint Structure and function, 2nd ed.. Philadelphia: FA Davis 1992;316-318.

95. Rothbart, B. Relationship of functional leg-length discrepancy to abnormal pronation. J Am Podiatr Med Assoc. 2006 Nov-Dec;96(6):499-504.

96. Eckoff, D., Johnston, R., Stamm, E., et al. Version of the osteoarthritic knee. J Arthroplasty 1994;9(1):73-79.

97. Huang, H., Keijsers, N., Horemans, H., Guo, Q., Yu, Y., Stam, H., Praet, S., Ao, Y. Anterior cruciate ligament rupture is associated with abnormal

and assymetrical lower limb loading during walking. J Sci Med Sport. 2017 May;20(5):432-437.

98. Golightly, Y., Allen, K., Renner, J., Helmick, C., Salazar, A., Jordan, J. Relationship of limb inequality with radiographic knee and hip osteoarthritis. Osteoarthr Cartilage. 2007;15(7):824-829.

99. Friberg, O. Leg length asymmetry in stress fractures. A clinical and radiological study. J Sports Med Phys Fitness. 1982;22(4):485-488

100. Ebringer, A., Rashid, T., Wilson, C., Ptaszynska, P., Fielder, M. Ankylosing Spondylitis, HLA-B27 and Klebsiella – An Overview: Proposal for early diagnosis and Treatment. Current Rheumatology Reviews 2006, 2: 55-68.

101. Finegold, S., Sutter, V., Sugihara, P., Elder, H., Lehmann, S,, Philips, R. Fecal microbial flora in Seventh

Day Adventist populations and control Subjects. Am J Clin Nutr 1977; 30: 1781-92.

102. Szeto, G., Straker, L., Raine, S. A field comparison of neck and shoulder postures in symptomatic and asymptomatic office workers. Appl Ergon. 2002 Jan;33(1):75-84.

103. Yip, C., Chiu, T., Poon, A. The relationship between head posture and severity and disability of patients with neck pain. Man Ther. 2008;13:148–154.

104. Diab, A., Moustafa, I. The efficacy of forward head correction on nerve root function and pain in cervical spondylotic radiculopathy: a randomized trial. Clin Rehabil. 2012;26:351–361.

105. Silva, A., Punt, T., Sharples, P., Vilas-Boas, J., Johnson, M. Head posture and neck pain of chronic nontraumatic origin: a comparison between patients and pain-free persons. Arch Phys Med Rehabil. 2009;90:669–674.

106. Diab, A., Moustafa, I. The efficacy of forward head correction on nerve root function and pain in cervical spondylotic radiculopathy: a randomized trial. Clin Rehabil, 2012, 26: 351–361.

107. Liu, XM., Pan, FM., Yong, ZY., Ba, Z., Wang, SJ., Liu, Z., Zhao, W., Wu, D. Does the longus colli have an effect on cervical vertigo? A retrospective study of 116 patients. Medicine (Baltimore). 2017 Mar; 96(12): e6365.

108. Ferreira, C., Bevilaqua-Grossi, D., Dach, F., Speciali, J., Goncalves, M., Chaves, T. Body posture changes in women with migraine with or without temporomandibular disorders. Braz J Phys Ther. 2014 Jan-Feb; 18(1): 19–29.

109. Watson, D., Trott, P. Cervical headache: an investigation of natural head posture and upper cervical flexor muscle performance. Cephalalgia. 1993;13:272–284.

110. Fernandez-de-las-Peñas, C., Pérez-de-Heredia, M., Molero-Sánchez, A., Miangolarra-Page, J. Performance of the craniocervical flexion test, forward head posture, and headache clinical parameters in patients with chronic tension-type headache: a pilot study. J Orthop Sports Phys Ther. 2007;37(2):33–39.

111. Chaves, T., Turci, A., Pinheiro, C., Sousa, L., Grossi, D. Static body postural misalignment in individuals with temporomandibular disorders: a systematic review. Braz J Phys Ther. 2014 Nov-Dec; 18(6): 481–501.

112. Tsunoda, K. Height loss caused by bent posture: A risk factor for stroke from ENT clinic - is it time to reconsider the physical examination? Acta Otolaryngol. 2011 Oct; 131(10): 1079–1085.

113. Lee, JH. Effects of forward head posture on static and dynamic balance control. J Phys Ther Sci. 2016 Jan; 28(1): 274–277.

114. Sonnesen, L., Petersson, A., Berg, S., Svanholt, P. Pharyngeal Airway Dimensions and Head Posture in Obstructive Sleep Apnea Patients with and without Morphological Deviations in the Upper Cervical Spine. J Oral Maxillofac Res. 2017 Jul-Sep; 8(3): e4.

115. Yong, M., Lee, H., Lee, M. Correlation between head posture and proprioceptive function in the cervical region. J Phys Ther Sci. 2016 Mar; 28(3): 857–860.

116. De-la-Llave-Rincón, A., Fernández-de-las-Peñas, C., Palacios-Ceña, D., et al. Increased forward head posture and restricted cervical range of motion in patients with carpal tunnel syndrome. J Orthop Sports Phys Ther, 2009, 39: 658–664.

117. Hyong, I., Kim, J. The effect of forward head on ankle joint range of motion and static balance. J Phys Ther Sci, 2012, 24: 925–927.

118. Alizadehkhaiyat, O., Roebuck, M., Makki, A., Frostick, S. Postural Alterations In Patients With Subacromial Impingement Syndrome. Int J Sports Phys Ther. 2017 Dec; 12(7): 1111–1120.

119. Renato de Souza Melo, Polyanna Waleska Amorim Da Silva, Souza, R., Raposo, M., Ferraz, K. Head Position Comparison between Students with Normal Hearing and Students with Sensorineural Hearing Loss. Int Arch Otorhinolaryngol. 2013 Oct; 17(4): 363–369.

120. Han, J., Park, S., Kim, Y., Choi, Y., Lyu, H. Effects of forward head posture on forced vital capacity and respiratory muscles activity. J Phys Ther Sci. 2016 Jan; 28(1): 186–189.

121. Bruno, A., Anderson, D., D'Agostino, J., Bouxsein, M. The effect of thoracic kyphosis and sagittal plane alignment on vertebral compressive loading. J Bone Miner Res. 2012 Oct: 27(10): 2144-2151.

122. Stovner, L., et al. The global burden of headache: a documentation of headache prevalence and disability worldwide. Cephalalgia 2007 Mar;27(3):193-210.

123. Smitherman, T., Burch, R., Sheikh, H., Loder, E. The prevalence, impact and treatment of migraine and severe headaches in the United Syayes; a review of statistics from national surveillance studies. Headache, 2013 Mar;53(3);427-436.

124. Vernon, H., Steiman, I., Hagino, C. Cervicogenic dysfunction in muscle contraction headache and migraine: a descriptive study. J Manipulative Physiol Ther: 1992 Sep; 15(7): 418-29.

125. Bogduk, N., Govind, J. Cervicogenic headache: an assessment of the evidence on clinical diagnosis, invasive tests and treatment. Lancet Neurol 2009;8:959-68.

126. Becker, W. Cervicogenic headache: evidence that the neck is a pain generator. Headache 2010;50:699-705.

127. Ulbrich, E., Schraner, C., Boesch, C., Hodler, J., Busato, A., Anderson, S., Eigenheer, S., Zimmermann, H., Sturzenegger, M. Normative MR Cervical Spinal Canal Dimensions. Apr 1 2014https://doi.org/10.1148/radiol.13120370

128. Diener, H., May, A. New aspects of migraine pathophysiology: lessons learned from positron emission tomography. Curr Opin Neurol, 1996 Jun;(3):199-201

129. Tajti, J., Szok, D., Pardutz, A., Tuka, B., Csati, A., Kuris, A., Vecsei, L. Where does a migraine attack originate? In the brainstem. J Neural Transm (2012) 119:557-568

130. Maniyar, F., et al. The origin of nausea in migraine-A PET study. The Journal or Headache and Pain 2014, 15.84

131. Sand, T., Vingen, J. Visual long-latency auditory and brainstem auditory evoked potentials in migraine: relation to pattern size, stimulus intensity, sound and light discomfort thresholds and pre-attack state. Cephalgia 2000 Nov;20(9):804-820

132. 2019 Encyclopedia Britanica

133. Lane, R. A critical review of selective serotonin reuptake inhibitor-related sexual dysfunction: incidence, possible etiology and implications for management. J Psychopharmacol 1997; 11: 72 ± 82.

134. Modell, J., Katholi, C., Modell, J., DePalma, R. Comparative sexual side effects of bupropion, uoxetine, paroxetine, and setraline. Clin Pharmacol Ther, 1997; 61: 476 ± 487.

135. Song, C., Korgaonkar, M., Armstrong, L., Eagles, S., Williams, L., Grieve, S. Tractography of the Brainstem in Major Depressive Disorder Using Diffusion Tensor Imaging. Published: January 21, 2014 https://doi.org/10.1371/journal.pone.0084825

136. Edelmayer, R., et al. Medullary pain facilitating neurons mediate allodynia in headache-related pain. Ann Neurol 2009 feb. 65(2):184-193

137. Brink, T., et al. Differential modulation of neurons in the rostral ventromedial medulla by neurokinin-1 receptors. J Neurophysiol 2012 Feb;107(4):1210-1221

138. Carlson, J., et al. Sensitization of pain-modulating neurons in the rostral ventromedial medulla after peripheral nerve injury. J Neurosci 2007 Nov 28;27(48):13222-31

139. Rosenberg, W., et al. Compression or the upper cervical spinal cord causing symptoms of brainstem compromise. A case report. Spine 1998 Jul 1;23(13): 1497-500

140. Breig, A. Biomechanics of the central nervous system. Some basic normal and pathological phenomena. Almqvist and Wiksell, (1960) Stockholm

141. Breig, A. Adverse mechanical tension in the central nervous system. An analysis of cause and effect. Relief by functional neurosurgery. Almqvist and Wiksell, (1978) Stockholm

142. Doursounian, L., Alfonso, J., Iba-Zizen, M., Roger, B., Canabis, E., Meininger, V., Pineau, H. Dynamics of the junction between the medulla and the cervical spinal cord: an in vivo study in the sagittal plane by magnetic resonance imaging. Surg Radiol Anat (1989) 11: 313–322

143. 14. Bakris, G., Dickholz, M., Meyer, P., Kravitz, G., Avery, E., Miller, M., Brown, J., Woodfield, C., Bell, B. Atlas vertebra realignment and achievement of arterial pressure goal in hypertensive patients: a pilot study. J Hum Hypertens 2007 May;21(5):347-52

144. Hulse, M., Holzl, M. Vestibulospinal reactions in cervicogenic disequilibrium. HNO 2000 Apr;48(4):295-301

145. Tuchin, P., Pollard, H., Bonello, R. A randomized controlled trial of chiropractic spinal manipulative therapy for migraine. J Manipulative Physiol Ther. 2000 Feb;23(2):91-5

146. Raczkowski, J., Daniszewska, B., Zolynski, K. Functional scoliosis caused by leg length discrepancy. Archives of Medical Science 2010 Jun 30; 6(3):393-398,

147. Perdriolle, R., Becchetti, S., Vidal, J., Lopez, P. Mechanical process and growth Cartilages. Essential factors in the progression of scoliosis. Spine 1993 Mar 1;18(3):343-9,

148. Stokes, A., Spence, H., Aronsson, D., Kilmer N. Mechanical Modulation of Vertebral Body Growth; Implications for Scoiosis Progression. Spine 1996 Vol 21, Number 10. Pp 1162-1167

149. Aronssson, D., Stokes, I., Rosovsky, J., Spence H. Mechanical modulation of calf tail vertebral growth: implications for scoliosis progression. Journal of Spinal Disorders, 1999 Apr; 12(2):141-6

150. Stokes, I., Aronsson, D., Spence, H., Iatridis, J. Mechanical modulation of intervertebral disc thickness in growing rat tails. Journal of Spinal Disorders 1998 Jun;1 1(3):261-5

151. Von Korff, M., Deyo, R., Cherkin, D., Barlow, W. Back pain in primary care. Outcomes at 1 year. Spine (Phila Pa 1976). 1993 Jun 1;18(7):855-62.

152. Deng, T., Lyon, C., Minze, L., Lin, J., Zou, J., Liu, J., Ren, Y., Yin, Z., Hamilton, D., Reardon, P., Sherman, V., Wang, H., Phillips, K., Webb, P., Wong, S., Wang, R., Hsueh, W. Class II Major Histocompatibility Complex Plays an Essential Role in Obesity-Induced Adipose Inflammation. Cell Metabolism, Volume 17, Issue 3, 5 March 2013, Pages 411-422.

153. Hales, C., Carroll, M., Fryar, C., Ogden, C. Prevalence of Obesity Among Adults and Youth: United States, 2015–2016, U.S. Department of Health and Human Services

154. Pawlak, D., et al (2004). Effects of dietary glycemic index on adiposity, glucose homoeostasis, and plasma lipids in animals. Lancet 28;364(9436):778-85

155. Eller-Smith, O., Nicol, A., Christianson, J. Potential Mechanisms Underlying Centralized Pain and Emerging Therapeutic Interventions. Front Cell Neurosci 2018 Feb 13;12:35. doi: 10.3389/fncel.2018.00035.

156. Segerdahl, A., Themistocleous, A., Fido, D., Bennett, D., Tracey, I. A brain-based pain facilitation mechanism contributes to painful diabetic polyneuropathy. Brain 2018 Feb 1;141(2):357-364. doi: 10.1093/brain/awx337.

157. Salas, R., Ramirez, K., Tortorici, V., Venagas, H., Vazquez, E. Functional relationship between brainstem putative pain-facilitating neurons and spinal nociceptive neurons during development of inflammation in rats. Brain Res. 2018 May 1;1686:55-64. doi: 10.1016.

158. Nigro, L., Donnarumma, P., Tarantino, R., Rullo, M., Santoro, A., Delfini, R. Static and dynamic cervical MRI: two useful exams in cervical myelopathy. World Neurosurgery 2017 Apr;100.474-479

159. Food and Drug Administration [Internet]. Silver Spring, MD. FDA Briefing Information for the February 10-11, 2014 Joint Meeting of the Arthritis Advisory Committee and Drug Safety and Risk Management Advisory Committee.

160. Bhala, N., Emberson, J., Merhi, A., Abramson, S., Arber, N., et al. Vascular and upper gastrointestinal effects of non-steroidal anti-inflammatory drugs: meta-analyses of individual participant data from randomised Babb M, Koren G, Einarson A. Treating pain during pregnancy. Can Fam Physician 2010;56:25, 27.

161. Nakhai-Pour, H., Broy, P., Sheehy, O., Bérard, A. Use of non-aspirin non-steroidal anti-inflammatory drugs during pregnancy and the risk of spontaneous abortion. CMAJ 2011;183:1713-20.

162. Nielsen, G., Sørensen, H., Larsen, H., Pedersen, L. Risk of adverse birth outcome and miscarriage in pregnant users of non-steroidal anti-inflammatory drugs: population based observational study and case-control study. BMJ 2001;322:266-70.trials. Lancet 2013;382:769-79.

163. Galm, R., Rittmeister, M., Schmitt, E., Eur Spine J 1998; 7 (1):b55–58, Department of Orthopaedic Surgery, Tokyo Medical University Kasumigaura Hospital

164. Bronfort G, Evans R, Kubic P, Filkin P. Chronic pediatric asthma and chiropractic spinal manipulation: a prospective clinical series and randomized clinical pilot study. J Manipulative Physiol Ther. 2001 Jul-Aug;24(6):369-77.

Dr. Calvin Hargis is a University of Tennessee alumni and a Magna Cum Laude graduate of Palmer Chiropractic College. Board certified as a chiropractic orthopedist and a neurofeedback therapist, he is a multi-patented inventor and father of four. Dr. Hargis maintains his practice, Warwick Brain and Spine Therapy, in Warwick, New York.

Made in the USA
Columbia, SC
13 September 2021